Radsresident

Radsresident

A GUIDEBOOK FOR THE
RADIOLOGY APPLICANT AND
RADIOLOGY RESIDENT

● ● ●

Dr. Barry Julius

ISBN-13: 9781544907970
ISBN-10: 1544907974
Library of Congress Control Number: 2017905652
CreateSpace Independent Publishing Platform
North Charleston, South Carolina

Dedication

To the underappreciated but not forgotten radiology resident

Acknowledgements

● ● ●

An undertaking such as this cannot be performed in a bubble. Numerous people have provided me with excellent material for the formation of such a book, not an easy endeavor. In particular I would like to thank the following individuals for their assistance and writings that have enabled me to compile this book (in alphabetical order): Daniel Choe, DO, Leonard Morneau, MD, Danny Nahl, MD, and Debbie Paciga. In addition, I would also like to thank my fellow Radiology Residency Program Director at Saint Barnabas Medical Center, Lyle Gesner, MD, for some of the inspiration for several of the articles and also for his tireless editing work. I greatly appreciate the sagely advice given to me about publishing a book by the great blogger and author, James Dahle, MD from the White Coat Investor.

It is also important to mention my family including Giora Manor, P.E. who provided me with great advice regarding the structure of the book and my wife, children, and dog (Otis) that gave me all the support and time needed to complete this work. And, last but not least, I would like to acknowledge the support of my radsresident.com website readers and radiology residents who are the reason for writing this book.

Preface

• • •

As an associate diagnostic radiology program director, I routinely enjoy giving advice to medical students, junior radiology residents, and more senior radiology residents about the less "scientific" side of radiology. You can often find me in the hallway or in my nuclear medicine reading room discussing radiology applications with medical students, teaching financial management 101, advising newer radiology residents, and mentoring senior residents for a career in radiology. Unfortunately, many times I have to dispel rumors about incorrect and outdated information that residents read on the web. Reliable resources on the web for these topics are sparse and scattered. And, even when there is a reliable source of information, it will use technical jargon or does not relate well to the radiology applicant and resident.

So, I figured this is an opportunity. With my background and interests, why not create a credible website with relevant information that informally addresses typical radiology resident concerns and issues on one centralized website? Who better to write and compile articles than someone intimately involved in day-to-day operations of residency? And, so began my mission to establish the radsresident.com website with useful, easy-to-read information for the radiology applicant and resident, not about the typical scientific radiology knowledge of images, but rather the application, lifestyle, financial, and career issues faced by those applying to residency and those training in radiology residencies.

Somehow over time, this mission has morphed into the form of this book. The individual chapters are articles from the radsresident.com website that have been edited for content and compiled into an organized logical format. In addition, I have selected the most useful and relevant articles and divided the articles into three sections: Applicant Advice, Resident Advice, and Resident Career Advice so that the articles are easy to find and readily accessible. Finally, since many residents have severe debt and only a rudimentary knowledge of financial issues, I have created an appendix containing additional chapters on basic resident financial advice. You can now have the best of the radsresident.com website in the form of a kindle document or physical book anywhere you want to go.

Along the way, many of the lessons in the articles were learned the hard way- by trial and error. This book will enable you to avoid those pitfalls of training and residency that may prevent you from having the best experiences possible. In addition, the individual articles will make your application process and radiology training more focused and successful. I wish I were so lucky to have some of these insights prior to beginning my training!

Table of Contents

Section 1: Radiology Residency Applicant Advice

● ● ●

CHAPTER 1

What To Look For in a Radiology Residency

● ● ●

FOR RADIOLOGY RESIDENCY APPLICANTS, THERE is no one perfect radiology residency program and not one size fits all. Each candidate has his/her own needs, wants, and learning style. And, each program has its own positives and negatives. The goal is to match the applicant with the appropriate program so that the positives of the program fit well with the applicant's needs. The negatives should be minor and not detract from the radiology resident experience.

My goal for today is to discuss the important ingredients for choosing a radiology residency. Some of these factors are not often discussed in a typical online overview of what to look for in a radiology residency program. So, I thought it was important to include them. Included in my discussion will be of greatest importance to least importance: residency culture/hierarchy, location/proximity to family/friends, insider intimate knowledge of a program, rotations/equipment/procedure volume, university vs. community programs, private vs. academic run departments, graduating resident fellowships, conferences, research, mentorship programs, and board passage rates. In the end, it is the entire experience of residency that is most important and will allow you to become a great radiologist. So, I will put it all together at the conclusion to help you to make a final decision. To help you make this decision, I have assigned an individual point score for each factor that you should record for each residency you are considering for ranking. At the end, you can add up the points and compare to the other residencies on your rank list and rank each accordingly.

RESIDENCY CULTURE (5 POINTS)

This is probably one of the most important factors to think about when choosing a residency, but it is also one of the most difficult to define. The difference between happiness and misery in a program first and foremost often lies with the colleagues that you have. No matter how great the overall "experiences" of a residency program, if you hate the people you work with, you will not want to come to work. On the other hand, if the program is marginal, but the people you work with are fantastic, the radiology residency will not be so bad.

The problem with using this factor for choosing a residency is that it is a moving target. From year to year, new residents are chosen and old ones leave. So, the residency culture that is there today may not be present tomorrow. However, the attending, technologist, and coordinator support structures of the residency often remain fairly similar. So, it is important to get to know not just the residents you meet, but also the leaders and purveyors of the program.

For that reason, in addition to getting a sense of the "happiness" of the residents, you will want to determine the structure of the residency leadership style. Some programs have prescribed processes for everything that happens at the program. Other programs have a more laissez-faire attitude. Some programs have one or two leaders at the top that act as "benevolent dictators". Others have each of the attendings with equal say over residency issues.

No one structure is "correct". If you are the type of person that needs a well-defined structure at all times, the hierarchical structure would be a better fit. On the other hand, if you like to create your own path where you define your own schedule, you may rather be in a program where all have an equal footing.

LOCATION AND PROXIMITY TO FRIENDS/RELATIVES (4 POINTS)

Over my years as associate program director, I have found how important it is for residents to have a social outlet. Although not a "resident related experience" per se, this factor can be just as important. Being near loved ones, family, and/or friends can make the difference between a terrible residency experience and a great one. A support structure can be just as important as the residency program itself. I find that the best residents have a healthy support structure outside of residency. Therefore, the location and proximity to loved ones can be an important factor as the residency quality itself. For instance, who would want to be in Manhattan, if your children/spouse are located in California? If asked by medical students, I will usually mention that they need to take location into serious consideration.

Insider/Intimate Knowledge of a Program (4 Points)

As a medical student, it can be extremely helpful to rotate through the department of a radiology residency program that you may want to attend. If you know the residents and attendings prior to starting a program, you likely already know many of the upsides and downsides of the residency programs and where "the skeletons are hidden" even prior to beginning. This can be worth its weight in gold. It can be very difficult to tell what the true nature of a residency program is like prior to starting a program. Therefore, having insider knowledge can really help you when you begin your residency because "you know what you are getting into". These residents often are some of the most successful because they have a distinct advantage of knowing the attendings, residents, and the hospital system, even prior to beginning their residency. This is a factor that should certainly not be dismissed.

Rotations/Equipment/Procedure Volumes (4 points)

I am lumping these factors into one conglomerate because it is important that the residency has all the resources that you will need to be comfortable at practicing radiology. If you are in a program where diversity of patients and patient volumes are sorely lacking, you are also going to be at a loss when you are out in practice and have not seen those cases in your area of practice. Likewise, if the radiologists in a program do not perform procedures such as arthrograms or your program doesn't have a 64 or 256 multidetector CT scanner for the interpretation of cardiac CTAs, you will certainly not feel comfortable performing these procedures when you are an attending.

So, it is really important that you make sure to search for a program that has all the necessary resources to allow you to learn all the imaging and procedure skills you will need to become a competent radiologist. Furthermore, as summarized in the later chapter, **Best Radiology Electives for the Senior Resident**, it is really important that you have the ability to do rotations in areas of weakness or interest during your residency because hiring practices are looking for residents that can do a subspecialty but also are competent in most areas of general radiology practice. So when you are on interviews or looking up information on the web, make sure to look into these factors. Once you have started a residency program without all the important resources to make a great radiology resident, there is no going back!!!

COMMUNITY VS. UNIVERSITY PROGRAMS (3 POINTS)

The incoming medical student tends to put more weight on attending a "university program" rather than a "community" program than is probably warranted. There are distinct advantages to both that many medical students do not realize prior to choosing a residency program. A large academic university program is not the right fit for all. So, what are the advantages and disadvantages of each?

The large academic university program tends to have a depth of resources in specific subspecialties and have several attendings that just practice in one specific subspecialty. The smaller community programs, on the other hand, tend to have more general radiologists that cross cover multiple specialty areas. So, as a resident attending a university program, you will get a more in-depth experience focusing on individual areas. As a community program resident, you will tend to get a more private practice and "real world" hands-on experience. So these programs should attract different types of radiology residents.

In addition, at community programs, you tend to have more accessibility to your attendings and will more likely work one on one with that individual. Also, if you have a specific need, it is more likely that it will be addressed personally without having to go through "bureaucracy" to get there.

At a large university program, there are more physicians that will intercede with direct attending teachings such as senior residents, visiting fellows, fellows, and junior attendings. There also may be larger bureaucracies that you may need to get through in order to obtain specific resources within your program. However, there may be certain electives and rotations that may not be available at a smaller community program, such as connections for abroad electives or other opportunities.

So, this factor should play a role in your decision. But, it really depends on the practice you want to have when you leave the system. One is not better than the other for all.

PRIVATE VS. ACADEMIC RUN DEPARTMENTS (3 POINTS)

This factor is often not mentioned or included as a factor in making a residency program decision. But having worked at private, hybrid, and academic programs, I really think it should be an important factor.

I completed my residency in the private/academic hybrid model and I found there were some real distinct advantages to this sort of residency program. We had to get through a specific number of cases each day to meet the appropriate caseload. In fact, it was a more "real world" experience that allowed me to hit the ground running when I started my first job. I was dictating loads of cases from the very beginning and had tons of experience by the time I graduated. This was very different from some of my more academic run department trained colleagues that I knew. Some of them had more difficulty with getting through lots of cases during the day and felt a bit more uncomfortable at their first community radiology job. It really made a difference in the long run for me, as it allowed me to become a more efficient general radiologist.

Academic run departments with attendings hired by the hospital emphasize different qualities. These departments may have more resources dedicated to teaching on a daily basis. For the resident interest in a pure academic job, it may be heaven!!! But, they may not simulate the real world. They can perseverate on a few cases for a long period of time. So, for the radiology resident that is interested in private practice, a residency such as this may not be the right fit.

CONFERENCES (3 POINTS)

All residencies are theoretically required by the ACGME to have at least one daily conference. But, not all conferences are created equal. Some programs have additional morning conferences. Others have the resident prepare for and present at interdisciplinary conferences. And, even others have residents prepare medical student teaching conferences. The styles and types of conferences can vary widely at each individual program.

Additionally, it is important to ask if the attendings regularly show up to give their conferences. Beware the program that has many sorts of conferences on paper, but in reality, does not actually have the number of conferences that they suggest.

The importance of the number and type of conference depends on the individual resident. Some residents learn better with didactic conferences and others benefit by hands-on direct radiology experience. So, the importance of this factor will vary with the individual applying.

GRADUATING RESIDENT FELLOWSHIPS (3 POINTS)

It is very important to check where the former residents have gone to fellowships. Are the residents not able to get into competitive subspecialties? Are they going to "no name" programs? Do the attendings at the institution have connections and networks with other fellowship programs throughout the country? These are questions that you should ask when you get to your residency interview or you should check online for this information. This can be crucial for getting your fellowship in an area and subspecialty that you are interested.

RESEARCH (2 POINTS)

For the academically oriented, research can be an important factor for selecting a radiology residency. For the community oriented, it is less so. But, when you look for jobs, having done some research implies an interest and commitment to radiology. So, it is important to have had some experience on your resume to get both the academic and private practice job. Therefore, research within an institution should play some role in your decision.

To make this assessment, it helps to get a list of the resident research output over the past 5 years. You can see what kinds of studies have been completed. Are there retrospective studies, case reports, or large prospective trials? Is each resident completing lots of projects? Does the program have research conferences to support the resident? These findings should help you decide if the residency has a serious program that encourages residency research.

MENTORSHIP PROGRAMS (2 POINTS)

Some residency programs have a dedicated teaching program that helps out first-year residents and gives didactic lectures. Others assign an attending mentor to the resident that is the "go to" person for all issues during their 4 years of residency. These are nice perks that when added to the other factors can be used to make a final decision.

BOARD PASSAGE RATES (1 POINT)

I am going to include board pass rates last because I believe that studying for the new core exam is more of an individual responsibility. Of course, you need to pass your boards, but I think that the overall residency experience is more important in the process of making you into a great radiologist than the board passage statistics. On the other hand, a radiology residency program should have the basic resources so that the applicant should be able to pass the exam. They should have learning materials and books as well as board reviews. There are many great residencies that have had lower board pass rates over the past few years, both large academic institutions and small programs. In the end, the examination is very different from the practice of radiology, but it is another hurdle to overcome.

Putting It All Together

There is no one factor that should make your decision to go to a specific program. But rather, the different factors should be weighed based on the individual applicant's needs and wants. So, add up the numerical point totals for each program next to each section and come up with a final score to create a final rank list for every residency program.

To summarize though, for most residents, I sincerely believe that you really need to take the residency culture to be one of the most important conditions for ranking a program in the residency match. And, location can have a great effect upon your happiness or misery during those 4 years. But, a great culture and location without adequate resources for training would certainly not be enough. So, be careful when you take each factor into consideration.

A great radiologist is the sum of one's experiences that often stems from radiology residency as the initial building block. Make sure that the foundation will provide you with the training you need to become the best you can be. It can be a difficult choice, but I hope I have been able to provide you with the tools you need to make that decision. Good luck with the match!!!

CHAPTER 2

Radiology Residency Night Float Vs. Standard Call- A Perpetual Controversy

● ● ●

BLURRY VISION SETTING IN; EYELIDS drooping just wanting to shut; difficulty communicating; impending malaise. Rarely would I have any chance whatsoever to lay my head down even once. The films would just keep on streaming in.

These feelings were typical on the first night of call of a 1 or 2 week night float rotation block or the occasional Saturday overnight calls that I would have to do every once in a while. I dreaded those days. But, it is still standard for most radiology residency programs, even now. It is almost impossible to not have at least a few overnight shifts like the one I just described.

At one point or another, many radiology programs and radiology residents have come up with different schedules and options in order to minimize this extreme fatigue. Some have instituted night float schedules. Others maintain a standard rotating call schedule Q4, 5, or 6. Some have long and short call schedules.

The choice to do one system or another is not so clear-cut. Many considerations have to be taken into account before pushing for a decision to have either of these systems prior to implementation. Although I tend to favor the night float system, since I remember it personally mitigated fatigue after the initial day or two of call when I was taking overnight call, the decision to have a night float program is probably not right for all programs.

So what are the factors that would lead one program to have a night float system and another to have a standard call system? Some of the issues that need to be addressed are the size of the program, attending coverage, resident preferences, program director preferences/department culture, number of nighttime studies, and the emergency department requests. Also, I will also go through the disadvantages and advantages of each system that will also allow a program to make a determination of which system is best.

Factors For Instituting A Night Coverage System
Size of the Program
The smaller the program, the less likely there will be adequate coverage for rotations during the daytime, let alone the nighttime. In fact, at many programs, a small residency cohort prevents the institution of a night float system. In a program with 3 or fewer residents per year, it may not be possible to have a resident out every night in order to be on call without severely compromising resident education. Also, it is possible that daytime obligations cannot be covered if a night float system is instituted.

Attending Coverage
Institutions with attending and/or Nighthawk coverage at nighttime allow more flexibility for scheduling of night float. In fact, some programs do not even need full-time resident coverage during the nights and may share call obligations with attending coverage. Therefore, it is significantly easier to institute a night float system for the residency program.

Resident Preferences/Culture
In some residencies, the radiology residents have instituted a night coverage system that may be based upon the preferences of the individual residents. Many residents are fully invested in a given system. If the system is

changed, there is a perception of "unfairness" because some residents may need to take more or less call than they would have in the old system. So, the night coverage system in place becomes engrained into the fabric of the residency program.

Also, scheduling may be set up to accommodate specific residency daytime programs. A nighttime schedule may be coordinated so that it allows the resident to maximize daytime educational opportunities. At some programs, that may mean either a standard cyclical call schedule and for other programs, it may mean a night float schedule.

PROGRAM DIRECTOR/CHAIRMAN PREFERENCES/DEPARTMENT CULTURE

At many programs, the leaders of the program, not the residents, institute the nighttime coverage. Therefore, the coverage may be based on the preferences of the program leadership. The program director or chairman may believe that a night float system or standard call schedule may be better for any given residency program. Or, perhaps there are coverage requirements that the department desires. In either case, it may not be a decision that is left to the residents.

NUMBER OF STUDIES

Perhaps you are at a residency program that is a level 1 trauma center with significant numbers of ER studies at nighttime. Some programs are so busy that they may need more than one resident or attending on call each evening. This may allow less flexibility to schedule a night float system since a program may not be able to accommodate the call coverage at nighttime.

EMERGENCY DEPARTMENT FACTORS

Emergency departments may have specific requirements for the radiology coverage at nighttime. Some programs may only want to have senior residents take call. Others specifically want attending coverage during the nighttime. Depending upon the demands of the emergency department, this may dictate the numbers, type, and the presence of residents or attendings on call. A night float system or standard call system may have to be based on the whims of the emergency department.

Advantages/Disadvantages of Each System
Night float

For most people, I personally think night float coverage for a week or two at a time mitigates fatigue the most. The body tends to get accustomed to the nighttime schedule over time and allows the resident to function better on call. Sure, the first few days can be tough because the body and mind have to adjust. But overall, the experience is much improved.

On the other hand, when you are on a night float system, the resident may lose touch with the "educational" aspects of the residency program. You miss daytime lectures and conferences as well as attending readouts for long periods of time. While the time spent on night float is important for training, it is impossible to receive all the benefits of daytime resident education. You may lose out on understanding the context of the images that you are interpreting. Education in this sense may also be compromised.

Standard Call

Sometimes a Q4, 5, or 6-day call schedule integrates better with a program than a night float system and allows the resident to get a better overall experience. The resident does not miss out on all the noon conferences and educational experiences that they would be missing over a long block on a night float.

The two big disadvantages to the cyclical call schedule: significant overnight fatigue and the "lost day". As I mentioned at the beginning, I always found it much more taxing to have an occasional overnight than a night float block, because my body never adjusted to the system. I think that this same issue can be extrapolated to most residents. In addition, the resident loses an extra day of residency experience every time he/she works because the resident is obligated to have a day off after call or "the post call day". This can significantly decrease the educational opportunities for the resident.

RESIDENCY CALL- WHICH SYSTEM SHOULD YOU CHOOSE?

The nighttime call is an important facet of every radiologist's education. Whether or not you have a say in constructing your program's night coverage system, you now realize that what works for one program, may not work for yours. The decision to have one or another system can be complex, but it is important to weigh each of the factors to come up with a final outcome. The key is to make the learning opportunity as pleasant as possible and mitigate fatigue. Hopefully, your prospective residency has chosen the most appropriate night coverage system for its needs!

CHAPTER 3

Cracking The Radiology Residency Application Code

● ● ●

TRUE INSIGHT INTO THE APPLICATION and interview process for radiology residency and fellowship is limited to most medical students and residents. The process can be clouded at times by misleading advice and rumors. Only someone on the inside can really understand what you need to know when you are applying for a radiology residency. Thankfully, you have come to the right chapter. I have looked at thousands of applications and interviewed hundreds of residents for positions in our program during the course of many years as associate program director. I am going to delve into the depths of the radiology residency application process and enumerate what you need to know.

THE APPLICATION

There are lots of ways to go through this. But I think the best way is to go through the different parts of the application from most important to least important so you don't squander your energy on the small stuff!

1. THE DEAN'S LETTER

There are few sections of the application that truly differentiate one applicant from another. Dean's letters happen to be one of those items. The reason for that: you will actually get comments from attendings, residents, nurses, technologists, and secretaries that may say something negative about an applicant. I can't tell you how many times we have parsed an entire application with glowing positives until we arrive at the Dean's letter. And, then we receive coded messages in the letter such as: was very shy during the rotation, but did see some improvement. Or, this resident was very independent but did not seek help when presented with a challenging patient care issue. And so on, and so forth.

Additionally, the Dean's letter may be the only document in the application other than the boards that compares the applicant to his/her classmates. Most medical schools have buzzwords indicating the resident's rank in his/her class. Each one is different, but typically it allows insight into which quartile the resident resides.

Ok, so you have your Dean's letter written in "stone". The institution administrators may say you cannot change the Dean's letter. But that is not true. Every medical student applying for residency should check his/her Dean's Letter prior to sending out the application. At some institutions, you can look at your letter prior to application time. If that is the case, you should certainly check it for any negative or questionable comments. And if possible, confront the department/person that wrote the comment and ask if they could redact or modify it. Obviously, if the writer is truthful, the person may decide to leave it in there. But an attempt should be made, as this one negative comment often makes the difference between high ranking, low ranking, or no ranking on a program's rank list. It is not infrequent that an admissions committee will obsess over one questionable comment. In fact, countless painful hours have been spent perseverating over these issues.

Other times, the institution may not allow you to look at the Dean's letter. But the school may allow your mentor or a faculty member to look at the document and possibly edit it for corrections. I can't emphasize enough how important it is to do this to increase your odds of being accepted to the residency of your choice.

2. The Boards/USMLE

The importance of the boards/USMLE for getting accepted to a radiology program is to assess the ability of a future resident to pass the radiology certification examinations. We have noticed a strong correlation between lower board scores and difficulty passing the new core exam and the old written/oral boards. Radiology board exams are notoriously difficult compared to many other specialties, so most programs take the USMLE score very seriously. The good news is that it is often used only as a baseline cut-off measure. Once you score higher than that baseline, it doesn't factor as much into the ranking equations. Failing and low scores, unless there are extenuating circumstances, usually place the application in the deny pile.

For those of you that are D.O. medical school applicants, I recommend that you take the USMLE in addition to the COMLEX examination. Many radiology programs are unsure of the significance of COMLEX scores and don't know how to factor the scores into the ranking equations/cutoffs. Applications with COMLEX scores alone may get thrown out of the interview pile entirely.

All this being said, there is some gamesmanship with the boards. If you have done very well in the step 1 boards, often times you may be able to get away with just sending those scores alone. In fact, you may want to delay taking the step 2 USMLE because those scores can only hurt you if they are lower. In addition, most programs look for/expect improvement from the step 1 to the step 2 boards, especially if the step 1 boards are borderline. So be careful and take the step 2 boards very seriously. Invest in a review course if you need to.

3. Research

Nowadays, research can be a significant factor for getting an interview in a residency program. What is the reason for that? Simply, the graduation guidelines for ACGME accredited radiology residencies have specific radiology research requirements for each resident prior to graduating. Knowing that a resident has completed multiple quality research projects means that a resident can work more independently to complete research projects within the program, reducing the burdens upon the department. Furthermore, radiology research may demonstrate significant interest in the field and provides an avenue for discussion at the point of the interviews later on in the process. Often times, we will look at an application and we will say, it's pretty good, but the resident hasn't completed any research. That may take the application down a few rungs.

Bottom line though. It won't take you completely out of the running for getting a spot but can be a big asset in some situations.

4. EXTRACURRICULAR ACTIVITIES

There are two big red flags when you are completing this section of your application: those people that have participated in every extracurricular activity under the sun and those people that have participated in almost nothing. A resident that participates in everything suggests that the person has a lack of focus, never investigating or accomplishing tasks in depth. On the other hand, a resident that participates in nothing but school tends not to be well rounded and may not have outlets to disperse their frustrations during their 4 years of training.

So what are some activities that impress the admission committee? : Interesting extracurriculars that show leadership potential, activities that demonstrate a depth of involvement, and activities that show an ability to handle stressful situations and function independently. Some of the special extracurriculars that stand out in my mind that meet these criteria would be a student that started a Subway franchise successfully from scratch and made it into a big business, a student that participated in the Olympics, and a student that was heavily involved in congressional lobbying. These are people that tend to climb the rank list higher because their extracurriculars were memorable.

What are some extracurriculars that don't really add much to the application? Those activities that everyone else does and do not suggest leadership potential. In radiology, those would include participating in a radiology club (Big deal!), participating in health fairs (Every medical student does it), and teaching inner city kids (We see it all the time as part of medical school curricula!) Not that these activities are bad, but they don't add much at all to your application. My recommendation is find some-thing you enjoy, hopefully, something unique, and stick with it during your 4 years of medical school training!

5. RECOMMENDATIONS

Admissions committees like to make a big deal about recommendations. You'll certainly hear that you need a great recommendation to get into a great program. But honestly, if you ask someone for a recommendation, it is unusual that you will find someone who is going to write you a bad letter of recommendation. It is obvious that students are going to ask attending physicians that like them. This statement brings us to one of the few ways that recommendations change the acceptance equation. It is a rare but major red flag to see a "bad" recommendation. It often means the resident that obtained the recommendation has a poor emotional intelligence quo-tient or couldn't find one attending that liked them- both major issues!!!

It is also the rare recommendation that raises the application within the pile to a higher rank or from no rank to rank. Usually, this type of recommendation comes from a well-known entity that wants the person in his/her own program or a close colleague that the radiology admissions committee implicitly trusts.

So, recommendations rank fairly low in the application influence equation.

6. THE PERSONAL STATEMENT

Finally, I would like to talk about the thing that medical students often perseverate on but has very little influence in the residency application process- the personal statement. The personal statement almost never helps an applicant and can occasionally hurt an applicant. After having read over a thousand of them, there are very few standouts. And, all of those that stood out were somewhat disconcerting. I still remember an essay that emphasized a dead rabbit and did not have any correlation to radiology whatsoever. I was concerned about mental illness in that student. That same person had the possibility of a radiology ranking immediately terminated!!!

My basic advice for personal statements is to be cohesive and relevant to your future career as a radiologist. Also, watch out for typos because typos suggest an inattentive personality, not a characteristic you want in a radiologist. Other than that, don't fret too much about this part of the application.

SUMMARY

Application for radiology is an arduous process with multiple pitfalls. Make sure you concentrate on those items that give you the most "bang for your buck" and will send your application higher on the rank list. Make sure to put particular emphasis on the Dean's letter. Check it if you can. Correct it if need be. Otherwise, make sure your application doesn't stand out too much. Don't be that student with marginal board scores, no research, with dull or no extracurriculars, with bad recommendations, and with a personal statement that stands out too much. If you follow these guidelines, you should get into a great residency, hopefully, one of your top choices.

CHAPTER 4

Radiology Personal Statement Mythbusters- Five Common Misconceptions About Radiologists

● ● ●

SINCE I STARTED WORK ON my radiology program's admissions committee in 2009, every year I notice a significant disconnect between the medical student impression of what radiologists do and the actual day-to-day work of the radiologist. The radiology <u>personal statement</u> is a shining example of this truth. In this chapter, I will debunk many of the myths espoused in the personal statements as to what we do on a daily basis (Just like the real <u>Mythbusters</u> (1)- this is going to be fun!!!). Let us begin...

WHERE'S WALDO?

Out of the thousands of personal statements I have reviewed, there are many that use the <u>Where's Waldo</u> (2) analogy in one form or another. In fact, if I see another personal statement with an analogy to Where's Waldo?, I will scream very loudly!!! But all kidding aside (I'm really not kidding!), this is one part of the radiology job that is not understood by many applicants.

So, what is it that a radiologist does? First and foremost- we read films and lots of them. Film reading heavily leans upon pattern recognition. And that is what we do. We use search patterns and compare our visual databank to the thousands upon thousands of images we have already seen. How does that differ from Where's Waldo? In Where's Waldo, the scenes typically differ on each page and you are expecting to find the same Waldo character in a sea of miscellaneous extraneous information or characters. For the radiologist, the scene is usually the same, whether it is a chest x-ray or a CT scan or even a Brain MRI. And, the findings can vary widely on any given film. You may find a pneumothorax or a herniated bowel loop or an infarct. However, you are not looking for one specific thing. You are looking for everything. This is very different from finding one Waldo, who is always going to have the same appearance. The analogy does not hold very well!

The One Fascinating Case

Often times, a personal statement will talk about one fascinating case and how that led the applicant to the decision of <u>choosing radiology as a career</u> (I am really sick of this conclusion!). Why does this point demonstrate so little insight into the day-to-day practice of radiology? Sure, every once in a while there is something really fascinating- perhaps it is a bezoar or a really rare tumor. And, sure it is great to perseverate on that case. But in reality, although exciting, these cases take up less than .01 percent of the work of the radiologist. You have to expect to pick up thousands of normals, normal variants, and common findings before picking up one of these rare zebras. So, when I hear that an applicant is choosing radiology for the one fascinating case, it really does not show a good understanding of our day-to-day work!

The Family Member Saved By A Radiology Finding

Sure, every once in a while the radiologist is the hero. We discover an occult aneurysm, the unexpected appendicitis, or the early breast cancer. And, maybe the radiologist has picked something up in your relative to save the day and has actually been credited. But in reality, how often does that occur? Not that often! In fact, it is pretty darn unusual. If you really want to save lives on a daily basis and get the credit, go into trauma surgery!!!

Radiologists, in general, have to be pretty humble because rarely are we showcased as an example of the medical profession for all to see. Usually, the doctors on display are the surgeons, internists, obstetrician/

gynecologists, or almost every other medical profession. Don't go into radiology to expect the glory of saving patients. We are usually behind the scenes!!!

The Diagnostic Dilemma

Many personal statements will describe a case where the radiologist went through a case and came up with an incredible differential diagnosis that was on target and well thought out. And, the applicant will point out that they want to go into radiology to make incredible interpretations. In reality, I also love a well thought out differential in an interesting case. Unfortunately, most cases are not in the category of the intriguing differential diagnosis. In fact, the final interpretations of cases are usually mundane and limited. So, don't expect to go into radiology to become the next House, MD every hour of every day!

The Isolated Radiologist

The last thing that we want to hear as radiologists is the amount of time that we spend in an isolated dark room, not speaking to others for hours at a time. Yet, many personal statements assume that we rarely come in contact with others and only plug away at the films. Although there are probably a few radiologists out there like that, it is usually the opposite. I can't tell you how many days, there is constant bombardment with technologist questions, physician consults, nursing issues, and more. Get your facts straight, before putting it in writing on a personal statement!!!

Busting Myths And The Final Truth About The Personal Statement

The good news: After all these false assumptions in many of these <u>personal statements</u> and out of the thousands of personal statements that have come across my desk, very rarely does one actually spur me to change a radiology residency applicant's disposition on the final rank list. In fact, I usually give these personal statements a pass because I understand it is difficult to comprehend what a radiologist does without having been through the experience.

On the other hand, if I had to give you one piece of advice as one of the main players in the application process at our institution, make sure you are not one of the chosen few that writes a personal statement that does influence our final decision. These are the personal statements with bizarre and sometimes scary thought processes and conclusions. The outcome of these weird personal statements is not usually positive! (meaning DO NOT RANK) So, stay away from the impulse to write something too unusual/different. We usually use the personal statement to weed out potentially psychotic behavior, not as a tool to make the final rank list.

So, as long as you don't write something too bizarre, I wouldn't worry about this part of the application too much. Just make sure to avoid the basic grammatical and spelling errors. And, most importantly don't try to rock the boat!!!

(1) http://www.discovery.com/tv-shows/mythbusters/

(2) http://whereswaldo.com/index.html#home

CHAPTER 5

10 Ways to Sabotage Your Radiology Residency Interview

● ● ●

AS RADIOLOGY ATTENDINGS, WE NEED to sit next to our radiology residents for hours at a time. We get to know your quirks, mannerisms, and other personality features for better or for worse. (Kind of like a marriage!) Interviews are a time to let that personality shine through. We want to make sure that you are a living breathing person with a soul. Can you speak understandably? Can you hold a conversation? Are you funny/witty? What's your personal hygiene like?

Interviews also confirm that you are the person you say you are in the application. Can this person be trusted? Is this person going to lie to his attending about a procedure or history? For these reasons, a significant amount of weight is placed on the interview even though the process is not perfect and does not always weed out the bad from the good.

Even knowing the importance of the interview process, many prospective radiology residents enter the interview unprepared and have the perceived emotional/situational IQ of a tomato. If that would be you, I would recommend you practice your advertising pitch numerous times prior to beginning the interviews. You need to be the greatest of actors/ actresses during the interview process if you want that residency job. Show us that you can handle the demands of radiology residency!!!

Throughout my years of interview experience, I have seen all sorts of applicant disasters during the interview process, usually related to unprepared applicants. Most of these catastrophes can be prevented with attention and practice. I am going to go through 10 real interview characters that have sabotaged their own application. I hope these scenarios will be instructive in the art of the radiology residency interview. DON'T LET ONE OF THESE CHARACTERS BE YOU!!!

1. THE LIAR

Our third interview candidate of the day walks into the room and shakes my hand firmly as we sit down to talk. He seems very focused and I enjoy talking with him. He starts talking about how he developed an organization that hires famous CEO guest speakers to come to his medical school and lecture on business in medicine topics. Wow, very impressive! The interview ran smoothly so I preliminarily give him high marks.

After the interview session, the selection committee convenes to review each of the applicants. Turns out, the application and the other interviewer had different stories. Upon review of the application, it says he was just a member of the organization's club. The other interviewer said he would only chauffeur the CEO to the meeting. Out of concern for the applicant's integrity, we put him in the do not rank pile.

Bottom line: Make sure to get your story straight. Your oral presentation and written information should all be aligned. The interviewers regularly reconcile everything together. You need to tell the truth and stick with the same story!!

2. SMELLY GUY

Prior to the formal interview procedure, we have a social interaction period with the residents to get to know the applicants. After most of the residents leave the room, we begin to hear some grumbling from the residents. So, I walk into the room and as I walk toward a particular applicant, a stench becomes stronger and stronger. Oh my God!! It smells pungent and I can almost taste it in my mouth. My impulse is to run, but I have to be cordial due to the circumstances. I am dreading the one on one interview process.

Bottom line: Make sure your hygiene is appropriate prior to starting your interviews. Appearances and "smells" are important!!

3. The Sleepy Man

My introductory lecture to our residency program starts and the lights begin to dim. I typically look at all the applicants in the room to keep the interest level high. But after 5 minutes of lecturing, I hear a loud freight train like noise emanating from the back row in the form of an applicant in a suit. My assumption is he is not interested in the residency program. Good applicant but low-interest level. We rank him toward the bottom of the list.

Bottom line: It is really important to get a good sleep the night before the interviews. Even if the applicant was only tired but really interested in our program, sleeping during the interview process shows a lack of interest and respect.

4. Ms. Robot

I warmly introduce myself to an applicant as she enters the room for the formal interview. Entirely devoid of emotion and empathy, she responds, "Hi" quickly. We sit down and the applicant immediately launches into this speech about herself without any voice inflection or changes in tone or speed. I have the sense she has done this a thousand times before. There is no "conversation-like" tone to her speech. No interactive quality. Is this the way she is going to behave when I have to sit with her for hours at a time? Even though her application was excellent, the applicant committee decides to give her a do not rank assessment.

Bottom line: Practice interviewing with others. Pretend you are having a conversation and interacting with your interviewer. Perceived personality is very important!

5. Shy Guy

The applicant walks into my interview room and introduces himself, but I can barely hear what he is saying. He stretches out to shake my hand. His hand feels cold, limp, clammy, and weak. The interview starts and I try to get him to respond to my questions, but it's like "pulling teeth". The answers last 10 seconds at most. I ask the residents who were sitting next to him in the conference room about the candidate and they say he didn't speak a word. No one was able to figure out his personality. Even though his application was OK, we felt we were unable to put him on the rank list.

Bottom line: You need to get over your fears and act and speak with confidence. It may involve practice, coaching, and/or psychological evaluation. If we can't figure out who you are during your interview, we are not sure if we want to sit next to you as a resident!!!

6. Mrs. Bizarro

Across from me in the interview area sits a pleasant appearing woman dressed appropriately. Everything seems fine until our conversation begins. Her eyes begin to bulge out. Smiles and giggles are inappropriately placed in the middle and end of sentences. Even though she answers my questions mostly appropriately, something is really off.

After the interview, we meet with the selection committee and the first thing I ask: what's with Mrs. Bizarro? All the members of the committee look at me and say, "We were thinking the same thing!!!" We quickly take her off the rank list.

Bottom line: Practice your interviewing skills in front of a mirror or tape yourself on an iPhone. You need to know that your expressions are appropriate for the interview context. This lady may have been an excellent radiologist but we sure would not feel comfortable having her sit next to us!!!

7. Not Quite Right Joe

It is toward the end of the interview and we start to talk about extracurricular activities and hobbies. The applicant proceeds to say that he was into cow tipping as a college student. And, one time the college dean reprimanded him for the activity. Automatically, mental bells start ringing.

Who would mention something like that in an interview setting? Why would someone want to do that to a cow? Off the rank list he goes!

Bottom line: We are not your friends in the interview setting. Do not release any information that could jeopardize your application and make you appear strange. We do not want any issues during residency that could cause probation, suspension, or worse!

8. The Guy all the Residents Hate

I am having a great conversation with one of the applicants. He tells me about some of his interesting research projects and hobbies. He seems to be a straight shooter and is very witty. We end the conversation on a high note with expectations that we are going to rank the candidate highly.

After our interview, we meet with the rest of the admissions committee. The admissions committee consists of the residency director, associate residency director (myself), a chief resident, and several other senior residents. We begin to discuss the candidate at hand. Every single resident states something negative like: "This guy was obnoxious"; 'He was chauvinistic"; "Really bitingly sarcastic". The directors are dumbfounded. The applicant is placed in the do not rank pile.

Bottom line: You need to play nice with all members of the staff, especially the residents. They have important input in the residency application process and interviews. The wrong statement can get you kicked off the rank list!!!

9. The Cell Phone Chick

I start giving the introductory talk to the applicants about the program. Every minute or two, I notice there is a woman looking down at her lap. Oh well... I continue on with my lecture.

An hour later, we meet for an interview and we shake hands. We sit down and I start asking questions. She seems a little bit distracted. Again her eyes continue to float down toward her lap every few minutes. All of a sudden, I hear a ring. She picks up the cell phone and says to me, "I need to get this". Obviously, she is not interested in our program.

Bottom line: Shut off your cell phone. You are here to interview for a job. It is a sign of disrespect to use your cell phone at any time during the interview process!

10. OPAQUE SAM

We parse through an applicant's resume and ERAS transcript. In the package, it states that the resident had a DUI arrest when he was a college student. So, the interview begins after some ice breaking small talk. Naturally, a DUI arrest is a big deal. It signifies that the applicant has potential to be an alcoholic and/or engage in risky behaviors. So, I anxiously pop the question: Tell me about what happened with your DUI arrest when you were in college? The applicant bluntly states, "It happened. It's over. I don't really want to talk about it further..." A moment of silence ensues.

Flash forward to the selection committee meeting. All the interviewers received the same response from the applicant. There was no response of remorse. No explanation for the event. Nothing. Our committee put the applicant in the do not rank pile.

Bottom line: Any negative events need to be addressed up front or else an admissions committee may perceive the applicant as hiding something significant, whether true or not. Don't be like Opaque Sam!!

SUMMARY STATEMENT

Interviewing is often about what not to do as much as it is what you should say. Make sure you are prepared for the interview day. And, don't be like our 10 catastrophic characters!!!

CHAPTER 6

The Post Interview Second Look- Is It Worth My Time?

● ● ●

EVERY YEAR AFTER <u>INTERVIEW</u> SEASON ends, there is a brief interlude until the rank selection list is submitted. You may wonder at this time- does it make sense to go back to a radiology program to take a second look? It may be a complicated decision and can depend on numerous factors. So, I am going to take a look at this issue from a program director's perspective and approach the problem by tackling a series of questions that will help you to make this important decision. Hopefully, it will be of some benefit to those of you that are involved in this process.

WHO IS MOST LIKELY TO BENEFIT FROM A SECOND LOOK?

From a residency director perspective, the ideal candidate for a second look at a <u>residency</u> program is a student that has already interviewed for which the admissions committee was unsure of its final disposition. Every once in a while, an application/prospective resident interview causes a stir among the committee. It may be the interview went really well, but the application quality didn't sync with the interview. Or, the <u>application</u> was really good but the applicant personality was questionable on interview day. Usually, it is some conflict in the committee evaluation process. These applicants can benefit the most from a second look because it may sway the admissions committee one way or the other after the candidate returns.

Second, the marginal/below average candidate that has been ranked but did not have many <u>interviews</u> would also be an ideal candidate to return for a second look. Some programs will rank their returning applicants a little bit higher for just showing interest by returning to the program. Usually, candidates don't return unless they are really serious about a program. A slight increase in the rank list can make the difference between matching and not matching.

Finally, the other ideal candidate would be the interviewee who felt he/she really didn't get the best impression of a program and wants to make a more informed decision on the day he/she will submit the rank list. Maybe the program director was absent. Perhaps you have a spouse that wants to remain in the area and you didn't get the best impression on the <u>interview</u>, but the location would be ideal. Or, maybe you really liked the people that you met, but you felt you didn't get to meet the key players in the residency program on the day that you interviewed. Whatever the case may be, the second look can help to reinforce that decision.

How Do You Know You Should Come For a Second Look?

Let's first begin by stating: The worst situation for the residency applicant and the program is to have an applicant that has already been placed into the "Do Not Rank" pile return for a second look. It wastes the applicant's time and money and the resources of the program director and staff. In addition, it may not make sense to the individual applicant to return depending upon other applicant factors. So, here are some criteria that may help you to decide if you are in either of these situations:

1. Did the interviewer suggest you come back for a second look? The program director will usually suggest returning for a second look if he/she is potentially interested in a candidate and think it may be of some benefit.

2. Did you get the cold shoulder during the interview process? Some interviews don't go well for multiple reasons. That will happen from time to time. Your instinct is probably correct if you feel that is the case. In this situation, it is probably not worthwhile to return for the second look.

3. How far down is the program on your rank list? If the program is very low on your rank list and you are a very strong candidate, it is probably not worth the effort to return for the second look.

4. Is it reasonable to travel to the interview site? Some candidates live very far away from the prospective residency program. If it is going to be disruptive to return to the program due to travel costs or significant inconvenience (maybe you are in the midst of your medicine sub-internship and can't miss a few days), it is probably not worth your effort.

HOW YOU SHOULD BEHAVE/PRESENT YOURSELF ON THE DAY OF THE SECOND LOOK?

The program director or interviewer that asks you to return for a second look will often tell the candidate "we would love to have you return for an ***informal*** second look". It is important to remember that there is no such thing as an "***informal***" second look. A second look is really a second interview day and needs to be treated as such. Wear your best <u>interview</u> clothes as you would have worn for your first <u>interview</u>. Be on your best behavior and be nice to **all** staff members just as you would have done for the initial <u>interview</u>. Remember... you still have not been admitted to the program and you are certainly not yet "one of the residents".

WHAT SHOULD YOU TELL THE PROGRAM DIRECTOR BEFORE YOU LEAVE?

There are certain buzzwords that have significance to the program director when meeting at the end of the second look day. The program directors and admissions committees take these words very seriously. So, be careful what you say. If you say the wrong thing, it may cause a different result than intended.

If you are truly interested in the program, you can say, "I will rank the program first." This is a very specific phrase and demonstrates a true intention to the interviewers. This fact can be verified on match day when you match at the program or do not match at the program. So, it is backed up by the facts. This truth will follow you from this point forward. If you ever decide you want to return to the community as an attending and you did not abide by your word, the program can potentially blacklist you!!! On the other hand, the phrase "I will rank your program highly" is a buzzword that means your program is nowhere near their first choice and you will probably match elsewhere. Some applicants do not realize this. So, be careful!

If you are still not sure after the <u>interview</u> day, it is appropriate to say, "I really enjoyed my second look at the program but I am still considering my decisions." The program director/interviewer will usually understand. When/if you do decide to rank the program first, you can always contact the program and let them know.

Final Thoughts About The Second Look

The second look can be an important part of the residency interview process. It can provide a slight edge to your candidacy and may be worthwhile if approached the right way. On the other hand, it may not be the right move for all applicants. So, weigh the facts and make a final decision. The <u>interview</u> process will be over before you know it!!!

CHAPTER 7

Radiology Residency And The SOAP Match

● ● ●

IT'S THE MIDDLE OF MARCH and every 10 minutes you are checking your email to see if you have matched in one of the most competitive specialties out there, maybe it was dermatology or radiation oncology. You can't eat or drink. Your mouth is dry. Suddenly, you get the dreaded email- "You have not matched for the 'blank' specialty in the regular match." *All these years of work and what do I have to show for it?* A wave of depression sets in. You want to stick your head in the sand.

Unfortunately, every year this scenario plays out. Each year the dynamics of matching in competitive specialties becomes harder and harder due to increasing numbers of medical schools/American MD graduates and stagnant American residency positions. (1) Not everyone gets his or her first choice of specialty during the standard NRMP initial match. Since this issue plays out for many radiology residency candidates, I thought it was important to give you some guidelines/tips about how to approach the issue if you are one of these residents.

WASH THAT FIT OF DEPRESSION AWAY

It is really important that you get into game mode. The SOAP process can be time-consuming and exhaustive from both an applicant and a program director perspective. But, in order to be a viable applicant, you need to move on and do what needs to be done. As an associate radiology residency director, one of my biggest turnoffs in the SOAP process is interviewing residents that are miserable and do not show a bit of enthusiasm for their new specialty choice. It is not the end of the world and it is a sign of mental toughness and grit if you can adapt to the new circumstances. Things don't always go our way!!!

If you are in this situation, it is also important to remember that you are not alone. There are numerous really qualified medical students that don't match. Often times the overall quality of the applicants is better than the initial match. So, don't take this as a sign that you are going to make a horrible resident. It's just not true.

THINK ABOUT YOUR OPTIONS

Residency is a long arduous process to enter a specialty that the applicant will work for the rest of his/her life. So, this decision should be well thought out and all applicants need to step back. Don't rush into applying to a specialty if you are not convinced that you have an interest. If you are not sure, there are other options such as applying for a transitional or prelim year and then reassessing the application during the year of residency. Only apply for the specialty of radiology if you are truly interested!

MOST APPLICATIONS IN THE SOAP ARE FROM DIFFERENT SPECIALTIES

We often get former applicants from matches of the most competitive specialties. Presently, these would be radiation oncology, dermatology, and some of the surgical subspecialties. Many years these specialties are completely matched with no slack. So, your two choices would be to reapply another year after completing a year of a preliminary medicine or surgical internship or to change specialties entirely. You take a risk either way. If you reapply, it is possible you may not match the following year as well unless there is a significant change in your credentials. On the other hand, if you decide to match in the SOAP for another specialty such as radiology, you may be matching in an area that you may or may not have a true interest. That hard choice simply has to be made in a very short amount of time. Significant self-reflection and analysis are really important at this juncture. Sometimes, the right choice is to apply to another specialty. I am a firm believer that we are underexposed to many different subspecialties during medical school and often times the best fit for a prospective resident is different from the specialty to which he/she initially applies. So, really think about the possibility of applying to a different specialty than you originally chose.

Also, don't worry if some of your recommendations, personal statement, and application are not geared toward radiology. The program directors usually understand the predicaments of the applying residents at this point. However, the applicant should come up with reasons for his/her newfound interest for radiology during the interview since enthusiasm for the specialty is very important. Make sure you really have a logical argument prepared for the phone or "in-person" interview for why you would be interested in radiology. It will go a long way toward securing a spot in a radiology program.

The Early Bird Gets The Worm

This is probably one of the most important factors in the residency SOAP match process. If you are not early on the draw, you are going to miss out on a spot. Make sure your application is submitted to your SOAP specialty of interest as early as possible. Often times, we find out about really good candidates only after the SOAP match has already been completed. Don't let that be you!!!

Try To Schedule Onsite Interviews If Possible

In the SOAP process, it is a major advantage to be able to match the face to the application. Although it is not always possible due to distance or other circumstances, if you are really interested in a position and you want to maximize your chances of acceptance during the SOAP process, an onsite interview really shows your interest and ups your chances of obtaining a spot. I always would rather deal with the known vs. the unknown entity. Usually, you simply get a better feel for the applicant when he/she is sitting in front of you rather than on a phone interview conversation. We have accepted applicants over the phone, but your chance of acceptance "in person" is simply higher. Try to physically get to the interview if possible.

Use Your Connections

Any connection to the SOAP match program of interest is of significant help. We really value the known vs. the unknown quantity when we are looking at SOAP applicants. So, if you have any connection to the program of interest, it will give you a leg up in the process. It could be a resident you met at some point earlier in your medical school training, a former mentor, or a friend of a relative. It doesn't matter. Any connection is often better than no connection. Use it!!!!

This Too Shall Pass

The SOAP process is short-lived but very stressful for all parties. Applicants and programs that did not match on the first try do often find a happy end to this story. Be enthusiastic, get past your depression, put the time and effort into the SOAP process, and you will often be handsomely rewarded. Don't take it seriously; be depressed about not matching into your initial specialty; or take a lackadaisical approach and you won't. Good luck with the match!!!

(1) http://www.usnews.com/education/best-graduate-schools/top-medical-schools/articles/2013/07/11/aspiring-med-students-face-growing-residency-competition

The Alphabet Soup of Residency Visas And The Radiology Alternate Pathway: A Guide For The Foreign Radiology Resident Applicant

● ● ●

DUE TO INCREASING GOVERNMENTAL BUREAUCRACY, static to slightly increasing numbers of residency slots, and increasing numbers of American medical student positions applying for residencies, it has become harder than ever to get a residency slot as a foreign medical student in the United States (1). That is not to say it is impossible to get one, but rather it is just significantly more difficult. Even though this is the case, since a large proportion of my readers are from foreign countries (approximately 1/3) and are interested in the mechanics of obtaining a radiology residency in the United States, I have decided to create a post about the world of visas and the radiology alternate pathway for ABR certification. Hopefully, this will be of some assistance to those of you with competitive applications and a burning desire to come to the United States for training. Also, I think it is informative and interesting for the United States residency applicant and radiology resident to understand what the additional requirements are for those that are applying from foreign countries.

In order to organize this post, I am dividing it into two sections. The first section will talk about the different types of visas with an emphasis on J-1 visas since this is the usual pathway that most foreign residents take to get a residency in this country. I will also briefly mention J-2 visas and go through some relevant information about H-1B visas and green cards/permanent resident status. The second part of this post will talk about the alternate pathway specific to radiology and what requirements are needed to satisfy the ABR if you have some foreign radiology experience and are considering not going through a standard four-year residency. Finally, I would also like to give special thanks to Debbie Paciga, our graduate medical education secretary, who was nice enough to take the time to share her vast knowledge on the topic of visas after many years of experience with numerous entering and graduating residents. Without her help, I could not have written this chapter!

Visas
J-1 Visas

A J-1 Visa is the most common type of Visa used by non-immigrant status foreigners for completing a residency program in the United States. Essentially, the J-1 Visa is an exchange visitor program for trainees from foreign countries. So, it is not expected that the J-1 Visa holder will become a permanent resident or citizen of the United States, but rather that the holder will be here for the limited time period of training.

Once the foreign graduate student has met the requirements of the ECFMG (Educational Commission For Foreign Medical Graduates), he/she can apply through the online system called The Physician Applicant System Access (OASIS) to obtain a J-1 Visa. However, the J-1 Visa requires a hospital sponsor in order to complete the application. The liaison between the teaching hospital and the ECFMG is called the Training Program Liaison (TPL) and this person accomplishes much of the work needed to obtain the J-1 sponsor. Typically, this person is a secretary or administrator whose responsibility it is to make sure that all the appropriate paperwork is submitted. This assigned person uses a system called The Training Program Liaison System Access (EVNet) on the EFCMG website to manage the application for the foreign graduate. Therefore, as a foreign graduate, you need to make sure that you are in constant contact with this person in order to complete all the necessary requirements for the J-1 Visa so that all the appropriate paperwork is submitted to this EVNet system.

So, what are some of the items that need to be submitted to obtain the J-1 Visa? You need to have a passport, a passport biography page, a curriculum vitae, a signed contract by the hospital and graduate student/resident with all the necessary information, the appropriate online filled-out forms (including the DS-2019 form- a form submitted by the sponsor), and of course all of the fees. Also, just as important, if you have a family that needs to travel to the country of the residency, you need to make sure that they have submitted a J-2 Visa which also needs to be approved by the sponsoring institution.

But alas, obtaining the J-1 Visa is not so simple as this... (It could never be that easy when it comes to anything that has to do with the State Department!) Each country has its own requirements for the applicant to be able to apply for a United States graduate education program. In fact, some countries have significantly limited the availability of these J-1 Visas. Each foreign applicant needs to obtain a statement of need from his/her home country embassy in order to be able to apply for the J-1 Visa. Some countries have severely curtailed the numbers of statements of need in order to prevent applicants from leaving their home country. The purpose of limiting the numbers at these particular countries is usually due to a lack of expertise or increased numbers of physicians needed in the applicant's home country. These countries do not want applicants to leave their home country and emigrate to the United States but rather want them to train and practice medicine in their home country overseas. Currently, some countries that limit the numbers of applicants the most to obtain a medical residency training J-1 Visa include South Korea, Sweden, and Canada. Then, there are countries such as India and Pakistan that tend to issue as many statements of need as warranted. Of course, this is a moving target and can change from year to year depending on a country's needs.

OTHER MISCELLANEOUS REQUIREMENTS AND ISSUES FOR THE J-1 VISA HOLDER

Once the J-1 Visa is obtained, there are numerous other requirements that the J-1 Visa holder needs to be aware of. For instance, the J-1 Visa holder cannot arrive into the country more than 30 days prior to beginning their residency. Sometimes, this can be a difficult issue since there is such a rush to get everything the applicant needs ready prior to beginning residency (housing, etc.).

Other recurrent issues include updating the J-1 Visa on a yearly basis with a new signed contract, obtaining recurrent statements of need from the home country of origin (sometimes the statements of need are time limited for less than the time of the residency program), and making sure to bring all the necessary documents when entering and leaving the country (up-to-date passports, diplomas, and so on...)

Applicants also need to beware of the legal system within the United States. The state department tracks illegal activities for residents with J-1 Visas on a yearly basis. Any conflict with the law can be a potential reason for the applicant to be sent back to his/her home country.

Finally, it is important to recognize that a research J-1 Visa is not the same as a J-1 Visa for a clinical residency. So, if you are a foreign national applying for a residency program, you need to obtain an entirely new J-1 Visa in order to start the program. (Whew, that's a lot of stuff to remember!!!)

H-1B Visas

So, what exactly is an H-1B Visa and how does it work for the residency applicant? An H1-B Visa implies that you are going to be working in a specialty field/occupation that has a need for a foreign worker that cannot be met by a United States resident. The H1-B visa holder is permitted to stay in the country indefinitely, different from the J-1 Visa holder.

Typically, the hospital needs to sponsor an H-1B Visa for an applicant in order to get the foreign graduate into one of its residency programs. In addition, the number of H-1B Visas is capped each year, making it more difficult to obtain one. It often costs the sponsoring hospital thousands of dollars to work on an H1-B Visa due to the necessary legal and processing fees. So, for these reasons, an H1-B Visa is an uncommon route for the foreign radiology resident applicant. At our institution, it has been only used for exceptional circumstances. One example would be an applicant that is already in a program in the institution but cannot get a J-1 Visa because this person has a D.O. degree and is from Canada. (Apparently, a D.O degree does not qualify for the J-1 Visa pathway). Since it is a rarely used method for foreign applicants to obtain a radiology residency, I am going to limit discussion on this topic.

Green Card/Permanent Resident Status

Finally, the goal of some foreign resident applicants is to declare permanent residency within the United States in order to remain within the country with a full-time radiologist position and with the possibility of eventually becoming a citizen. The United States lists several mechanisms of obtaining a Green Card including via job offers, investing in enterprises, and self-petition (typically an individual of extraordinary ability). Many applicants will often get their green card once they have graduated from a residency program and have been accepted for a permanent radiologist position in the United States. At that point, the employer is required to file a petition for the employee so that he/she can undergo the application process and the applicant needs to fill out the appropriate paperwork. Usually, this process occurs only after the J-1 Visa is no longer active.

One other pathway to obtaining green card status (2) includes finding a position in an underserved area for a period of time, usually 5 years. This applies to not only primary care physicians, but also specialists as well. But again, it is usually completed after the radiology residency has ended.

The Radiology Alternate Pathway

In a past response to a question from a potential foreign applicant in the "Ask The Residency Director" section on my website about the alternate pathway (3), I briefly went over some of the requirements for the foreign radiology applicant to obtain ABR certification. The question asked about applying outside the typical route of a four-year qualified ACGME radiology residency based upon the applicant's previous radiology experiences. This process is called the Radiology Alternate Pathway. According to the ABR policy(4), the applicant can satisfy the requirements only at institutions with an ACGME-accredited radiology residency training program. The applicant needs to have 4 years of <u>continuous</u> work in the capacity of a "resident, ACGME accredited fellowship, non-ACGME accredited fellowship, or faculty member". In addition, the candidate must also have "4 months of clinical nuclear medicine training." The nuclear medicine training needs to be dedicated though the applicant can get the training at an affiliated institution if that is available.

The challenge for the foreign radiology applicant is to find a program that is willing to recognize previous foreign training and accept him/her for a slot in one or more of these programs over a four-year period. Many programs are not willing to make an obligation of four years of employment in a mixture of residency, fellowship, or faculty positions and will require the applicant to go down the standard pathway of radiology residency. That is not to say it is impossible. But rather, it is not common and represents the exception rather than the rule.

Final Thoughts

Applying to radiology residency and performing well in a radiology residency program as a United States citizen can let alone be challenging. Add to that the issues that arise from migrating to a new country and I can only imagine the additional difficulties that foreign applicants face applying to and attending radiology programs within the United States. There are certainly numerous hurdles and hoops for these applicants. But for those with the desire, ability, and grit/determination, it is still certainly possible to go through the process of getting a visa and obtaining a qualified residency spot or spot in an alternate pathway program. If this is your life's desire, don't let these hardships dissuade you!!!

(1) http://www.medscape.com/viewarticle/857443

(2) https://www.uscis.gov/green-card/other-ways-get-green-card/green-card-through-physician-national-interest-waiver-niw

(3) http://radsresident.com/2017/01/08/how-to-complete-the-abr-alternate-pathway-as-a-foreign-physician/

(4) https://www.theabr.org/sites/all/themes/abr-media/pdf/PWIMG_DRandSubCert.pdf

Helpful Websites For The Foreign Medical Graduate

ABR Alternate Pathway Information- https://www.theabr.org/sites/all/themes/abr-media/pdf/PWIMG_DRandSubCert.pdf

ECFMG - http://www.ecfmg.org/evsp/application-online.html

Governmental Green Card Website Information- https://www.uscis.gov/greencard

Governmental J-1 Visa Website Information-https://j1visa.state.gov/basics/common-questions/

Governmental J-2 Visa Website Information- https://j1visa.state.gov/basics/j2-visa/

Governmental H-1B Website Information- https://www.uscis.gov/eir/visa-guide/h-1b-specialty-occupation/understanding-h-1b-requirements

Section 2: Radiology Resident Advice

● ● ●

CHAPTER 9

How To Make A Good Impression As A First Year Radiology Resident

• • •

IT MAY BE YOUR FIRST day, your first month, or maybe you've started residency several months ago. Perhaps, you want to make that great first impression on your program director or maybe things are not going as well as you might have liked during your first year so far. Having worked with numerous first-year residents rotating in and out of our residency and having had a full four years of residency behind me, I have learned the ingredients you will need to make a great first-year resident. As a former resident, I wish I had a list of tips on how to start my radiology resident experience on the best footing possible. Well, now it's here... I have a list of 12 ways you can improve your radiology residency experience starting out in your first year of your diagnostic radiology residency program. I will give you examples of what not to do (these scenarios are real!) and then explain how to make the best of each piece of advice. To all- ENJOY AND HEED THIS ADVICE!!!

1.BE ENTHUSIASTIC

On your first day of radiology residency, you walk into the reading room for the first time and you are nervous and hesitant. You begin to yawn, mouth wide open. There is an attending sitting in the corner about to read films. You slink back and worm your way into a corner. You don't introduce yourself for fear of disturbing the attending radiologist and you start talking to your resident colleagues. Is that a way to start your career? By all means, NO!!!!

My words of advice: Always make sure to put on your best face forward toward your staff. What does that mean? Well, it's pretty much common sense. Always introduce yourself. Always ask how you can help. Always volunteer to participate in a readout or procedure. You really have only one chance to learn the things you need to know prior to practicing as an attending and that way is RADIOLOGY RESIDENCY. Make it the best learning experience you can and that involves going that extra mile to show your enthusiasm/interest.

2. Be On Time

You straggle into the reading room and it's 10 o'clock AM. When you see your attending reading out films, he pauses for a moment. You decide to say, "When can we start reading out together?" The attending looks at you with a confused quizzical face. He is thinking *I was supposed to have a resident today?*

My words of advice: When you arrive in the morning always let your attending know that you are the resident for the day and if you have to step out for a few moments let him/her know that you need to leave for whatever reason. It is a sign of respect to let your attending know that you are going to be there to help out, learn, dictate, and ask questions. It will go a long way to establishing a rapport between yourself and your residency staff!

3. Be Nice to Everyone

It's your first day and you walk into the residency coordinator's office and you sit in her chair, never having seen or met her. You start playing games on her computer. The coordinator walks into the office and stares at you and is thinking: who the heck is this guy?

My words of advice: Make sure when you are starting out you are nice to everyone!!! I don't care if it is the residency coordinator, janitor, technologist, attending, a fellow resident, or nurse. We are all part of the same team and we always hear about our resident's behavior, good or bad. In fact, as residency director, we get 360-degree evaluations that involve reviews of the residents from potentially all these sources and more. I can tell you that if you want to destroy your reputation as a resident, the worst thing you can do is be inappropriate to any of our team members, especially the residency coordinator!!!!

4. DRESS APPROPRIATELY

You are upstairs on the floors in a t-shirt and ripped jeans and id badge in your back pocket going through the list of patients to consent. In your morning haze, you stumble up to the door of the 3rd patient with informed consent in hand. You introduce yourself to the patient and she gives you that look- *who are you really and what are you doing here?* You go through your pat explanation of the procedure, the risks, and the alternatives. The patient warily signs the consent form. Great! The last consent of the morning... Later that afternoon the program director calls you into the office. Turns out, the patient was the wife of a hospital executive and called the emergency hotline. The program director now has two complaints about this resident, one from the patient's husband and another from the doctor in the hallway. Both are furious because they weren't sure who you were and felt really uncomfortable confronting you. The program director states, "Go home and change immediately!"

My words of advice: Always make sure you look like and play the part of a physician. Some patients and physician are easily offended by an inappropriate appearance/uniform. In our world, we are a service-oriented profession and appearances fortunately or unfortunately lend credence to your skills, personality, and the department. Please make sure to represent your department in the best light!

5. Play the Role of An Attending From Day One- Take Responsibility for Your Patients and Department

You roll on into the nuclear medicine department and arrive at the department early. You briefly look at the list of patients in the computer. There is a bone scan and a gallium scan that have not been read. You think to yourself, I know those topics really well and it would be much more productive to read a nuclear medicine book on a new topic that I don't know much about. As you are waiting for your attending to arrive, you pull out your book and begin to read about nuclear medicine. The attending walks through the door a few minutes after you started to read and says "Have you looked at the cases from last night?" You reply, "I was hoping to get my reading done for the day. Didn't get a chance to look at the cases."

My words of advice: When you are on any service, the best way to learn radiology is to read lots of cases. You may know a given topic well, but the only way to differentiate normal from abnormal is to read thousands and thousands of cases in different contexts, an activity that you cannot learn from reading a book. And the only way to get that experience is to look at the cases every day. Take an active role as if you are an "attending". Radiology is not a spectator sport!

6. Be Knowledgeable

You are on your second week of your first CT rotation and you sit down with the CT attending to go over the day's work. The attending goes through each of the cases slowly and finally happens upon an abdominal CT scan. You stare at the images and he asks you what this ovoid cystic density structure is just inferior to the liver. You blurt out, oh that's easy… it's the aorta!!! Your attending begins to shake his head slowly and becomes silent. He doesn't say much for the rest of the day.

My words of advice: There's an old radiology adage. The difference between a bad, ok, good, and great radiology resident is the amount you read every night. A bad resident doesn't read. An ok resident reads 1 hour a night. A good resident reads 2 hours a night. And, a great radiology resident reads 3 hours a night. Don't be that bad radiology resident! When you start, I encourage you to read a lot, especially emphasizing the basics and anatomy!

7. Read a Lot, but Make Sure to Study the Images

It is your first day on the new chest film rotation and you just finished reading an entire textbook on chest radiology. You start looking at the cases with your attending and you figure you will try to impress him with your deep knowledge of the findings associated with sarcoidosis. So, you start going through a small presentation about your newfound knowledge based on the textual information. After your serenade, he starts to look at the first few cases of the day and then pauses as he arrives at the third case of the day. He asks, "What do you think about this chest film in front of you?" You stay silent as you search the film up and down, left and right. Nothing seems to register as abnormal on the film. Your attending points out a large opacity obliterating the vessels behind the heart and obscuring the left hemidiaphragm. He then asks, "Where the opacity is located?" You realize that you have read tons of information on pneumonia but never looked at the pictures so you couldn't identify the location based on a mental reference point. Your heart sinks as you realize you have more reading to do...

My words of advice: Reading a radiology text is very different from reading an internal medicine book, a novel, or other sorts of written information. The most important features of a textbook are usually the pictures and captions below the pictures. It behooves the resident to concentrate on these films, often more than the text itself. It is important to understand and remember the disease entities, but radiology is most often about the images!

8. If a Radiology Attending Asks You a Question, Always Look Up the Answer

So it's the end of the day and you are sitting with your favorite attending. For the few days that you have worked with her, she has a habit of teaching interesting topics while she is taking cases. It feels like you just read an entire book without even touching a page. She enthusiastically asks you a question about a patient with breast cancer. She says, "I wonder what a sclerotic metastasis would look like on a PET-FDG scan? Maybe you can look it up and we will go over it tomorrow."

So you go home exhausted and fall asleep slumped over your computer, without even getting a chance to read a word about the topic. You get up in the morning and realize you are running late. You grab your stuff and get to work barely on time. You run into the reading room in a sweat. Your attending is about to sit down at her workstation. And she says, "Did you look that topic up for me?" You don't really have a satisfactory answer. For the rest of the day and for weeks afterward, she barely spends time on her cases with you. You've lost many opportunities to learn with your mentor.

My words of advice: You sow what you reap! When someone, specifically a radiology attending, takes the time out of the day to teach and goes over cases with you out of his/her own free will, it is important to pay back that person with attention, diligence, and care. There is nothing stronger than under appreciation of an attending's time to change the willingness of a teacher to teach. Remember, most radiologists are not paid for their time with their residents. Teaching emanates from the good will of the staff!

9. ALWAYS GET A GOOD HISTORY.

It is late in the day and you are about to try to read the last hepatobiliary scan of the day. But you have to do it quickly because you need to get home to your family. So you peruse the one-word order on the top of the dictation page that is often filled out by a clerk or a nurse without any real history whatsoever. It says pain. So you start reading and dictating the case promptly for the attending with that one-word history. In a few minutes, you are done. You walk back to the reading room and begin to go over the case with your attending. Subsequently, he opens the case, looks at your history/dictation and begins to look at it as the surgical team walks by to get the radiologist's interpretation. The surgeon asks, "What do you think?" The radiologist replies, "With a history of pain, it look like the gallbladder fills nicely without findings to suggest cholecystitis". The surgeon responds curtly, "We just took out the gallbladder!!"

My words of advice: Always take the time to get a great history. Residency is a time when you actually have the time and wherewithal to gather all the information. I can guarantee you this scenario and similar situations happen all the time. You will get burned many times without a good history. So, avoid the inevitable, take your time, and always get all the necessary information!!!

10. ESTABLISH A SEARCH PATTERN FOR ALL MODALITIES

The attending of the day sends you out of the room to read a new CT scan of the abdomen in a patient with right lower quadrant pain to rule out appendicitis. So you look through the CT scan quickly and ramble into the Dictaphone about the case. Your eyes move here and there without any specific pattern. Finally, you see some terminal ileum wall thickening and put in your impression- findings suspicious for terminal ileitis/inflamma-tory bowel disease. Happily, you trot back to your radiology attending to go over the case. Within 10 seconds, your attending says, "You missed the 4 mm obstructive stone in the right ureter!"

My words of advice: Believe it or not, almost every experienced radi-ologist has a rigorous search pattern and mental checklist on every case so they don't miss any findings that may be relevant to patient care. You might not know they have a search pattern/checklist because they have been doing it for so long and are so quick at reading a case. But, I can guar-antee you will miss plenty of important findings if you do not go through an organized approach to looking at a film. It happens all the time!!!

11. ALWAYS CHECK FOR PRIORS

The radiology attending just left the service for the day and you are now on call for the night. The emergency department continues to call the nuclear medicine department every 10 minutes to get the result. Annoying, isn't it? It is time to give a stat interpretation of a pulmonary V/Q scan. So, you look at the scan and the associated chest film and you see 3 large mismatches without corresponding findings on the chest film. You call the ER and tell them the scan is positive for pulmonary embolus. You feel good because you think you made the right call for sure. The next morning at readout your attending starts to look at the case. He notices that there is a prior scan that you didn't compare. It looks exactly the same. His interpretation- no findings to suggest new pulmonary embolus... He says, "Call the ER right now to make sure the patient doesn't get more anticoagulants." You feel like an idiot for giving bad patient care!

My words of advice: I can't emphasize enough how important it is to compare priors. There are so many times that priors will bail you out and make the difference between shoddy and really good patient care. If you want to be a resident star, always make a concerted effort to check for prior studies!

12. LEARN ABOUT THINGS THAT CAN KILL A PATIENT OR ARE COMMON FIRST. ZEBRAS CAN USUALLY BE LEFT AT THE ZOO!

You are taking your first independent call and start to look at your first ultrasound of the evening. It is a 2-year-old pediatric patient with right lower quadrant pain. You see a target like structure in the right upper quadrant. You just recently read a large text and saw a case of Henoch Schonlein Purpura affecting the bowel and it happens to look just like it. Your differential reads *Bowel thickening from Henoch Schonlein Purpura* before anything else. Ten minutes later the pediatric surgery team trots up the stairs toward your workstation and says, "What are you talking about? We were just looking for a large bowel intussusception!"

My words of advice: Stick to the most common two or three items within the differential diagnosis. You will often be right more than not. Like I said, zebras can usually be left at the zoo!!

SUMMARY

I'm sure almost all of you want to make your best impression on the staff that you are going to work with for 4 years. One or two mistakes toward the beginning of your stay can make your life very difficult for the duration of the residency. It is very easy to leave the wrong impression on the staff. To simply avoid these gaffes, I highly recommend you follow these rules. Don't be the brunt of your residency's jokes!

CHAPTER 10

Dictating- Tips For The Radiology Resident

● ● ●

DICTATION IS A TOPIC THAT is rarely touched upon in radiology but is extraordinarily important. In a radiologist's 30-year career, he/she may dictate over 360,000 reports (assuming 12,000 cases per year for 30 years). In today's world, it is mostly the dictation that spurs clinicians to act on their patients. Out of 100 cases, only a few are acted upon due to other circumstances such as conversations with a radiologist or by interdisciplinary conferences. These are the exception rather than the rule. Just like a manufacturing company that creates automobiles, dictations are the end product of the radiologist's service. After all is said and done, it is all that is left in the medical record after we are gone.

It is true that there is a "steep learning curve" for the radiology resident, meaning that there is a rapid incorporation of the techniques of dictation. Much is learned after the initial year of training. But it is only after years and years of experience that the dictation is fine-tuned to the point that the dictation has its maximum utility for physicians.

What are the differences between a radiology resident/newly minted radiologist and a seasoned radiology attending's dictations? Well, certainly there are always exceptions to every rule. But for the most part, when you look at the resident or new radiologist's dictations, you see a conclusion that is more verbose and a comments section that contains more impertinent findings. And, that perfectly makes sense because new physicians are putting their feelers out to get a sense of what is truly important for the clinician. Most seasoned radiologists already know this information innately from years of practice.

For residents, it is assumed that they will know how to dictate appropriately after a short period of time and that a radiology resident will just learn to dictate by osmosis. But, it is helpful for the resident to have some guidelines to make the transition easier. So, first I am going to discuss a little about templates for dictating. Then, I will give you some guidelines for each part of the dictation: the history, the technique section, comparisons, comments, and the impression. And finally, I will talk about the use of structured and prose dictations.

TEMPLATES:

When I was a resident just starting out, I remember we had a booklet of templates for all sorts of commonly used dictation types for residents. We would carry around this book during our first days of dictation and would dictate the information to the secretaries upstairs. Today most institutions use dictation/voice recognition software, but the template concept is similar. In fact, it is easier than ever to gather templates from other radiologists to be used for dictation when you are starting out. However, this sometimes complicates things because you may have many different types of templates to choose from for the same type of dictation. My recommendation is to find the best template for a given type of study and to stick to this one type of template when you are starting out. Sure, there will be radiology attendings that insist you use their templates for a given report. That is fine. You should certainly abide by your attending's wishes because in the end, it is his/her report. Overall, just try to be consistent. The more you use a given template, the more likely you will be to remember all the items that you need to include in a dictation.

Even as a seasoned attending, templates are still extremely useful. Why? They save time and I typically still use them as a checklist to make sure I have looked at all the different organs and physiological systems within the study.

But there are definite pitfalls to using a template. Be very wary... The biggest problem: you may forget to take out the pertinent findings embedded in the template. I've seen many reports go out with something like the following statement in the comments section: *The kidneys are normal* because it is the embedded information in the template. However, when you look at the beginning of the comments section and the impression, they say *there is a cystic mass in the kidney.* These inconsistencies not only confound the clinician, leading to phone calls but also can be medically and legally ambiguous and potentially dangerous. So always make sure to check your work twice before the dictation is signed off/completed.

Histories/Priors:

What needs to be placed in the history has significantly changed over time. When I first began my radiology residency, histories were initially expected to be a one or two-word blurb about the patient's condition. Now, with all the new regulations, accreditation bodies, and ICD-10 codes, the histories need to be longer in order to be fully reimbursed for a study. In fact, our billing managers recommend putting as much relevant data as possible in the history in order to ensure that the study is fully reimbursed. One example: When I first started it was frowned upon to put the age of the patient in the dictation history. Now, if I don't put the age of the patient in my cardiac nuclear medicine dictations, the reports cannot be sent to the accreditation body, for our hospital nuclear medicine department to continue accreditation. So, try to put in as much relevant/appropriate data as possible in the history to ensure the study is fully reimbursed and can be used appropriately. In addition, more history can also sometimes be more helpful for the clinician and can assist in formulating an appropriate conclusion to the clinical question.

It is also very important to put relevant information from prior studies in this section. Often times, residents will put this information in the body of the report. It really is not the place for the history. You can refer to the history from the body, but keeping the history in the body of the report can confound the clinician as to which data is from the current report.

TECHNIQUE:

The technique section is the stepchild of the dictated report. It is often times ignored by the clinician and the radiologist reading the dictation. But on occasion, it comes in very handy and should be reported accurately by the dictating physician. For instance, you may say *there is a 5mm axial slice thickness on CT scan.* If it happens to be you didn't see a pulmonary nodule on that study and the next study has a slice thickness of 2 mm, it may be that the pulmonary nodule was really present on the prior study but was not visualized because of the differences in technique. If this data is not correct, it can confound the clinician, the radiologist, or the report. So do not ignore this section and be very diligent with dictating the technique accurately.

Also, don't assume that the template technique is always correct. Many times residents and attendings alike will perform a fantastic dictation and then I look back at the technique section. It is totally wrong. The standard technique template format should have been changed. This error happens more often than physicians realize. Make sure to pay attention!

COMPARISONS:

There is some variability in the placement of this section. I tend to state comparison is made to the previous study dated *blank* at the beginning of the comments section. Others will make this into a distinct section. Regardless, it will make your comments and impression much easier because the reader will always know which study you are referring to for comparison when you state something is worse, better or improved.

COMMENTS:

The comments section is the place where the radiologist can "go to town". Here is the place where all the pertinent negatives and positives belong. Be detailed and specific, especially as a radiology resident. Describe the findings well. Make sure to put in locations, size, morphology, density, and so on. If you see an important finding, it is also a good idea to put in the slice number in the dictation. I have found over the years, it makes it much easier for the attending radiologist to find the abnormality that you are reporting, especially in the case it is subtle and may be hard to find.

One of the issues that confound the novice: should you put in the differential in the comments section or only in the impression section? I recommend stating the relevant findings in the comments section and then giving the expanded differential in the comments section based on the relevant findings. You can also state the reasons why you think your final diagnosis is what it is. That same information can be honed and tightened in the impression section later.

Again, be careful with using templates. Many times we will see inconsistencies in the report because standard template statements are left in the dictation. Make sure to erase the standard statements if you make a finding that is different from the standard normal template. Be very careful. Remember the report is a legal document and can be used against you in a court of law!!!

IMPRESSIONS:

The impression is the standard bearer and the central representation of the quality of the report. It is the place that should contain the information that is most pertinent to the clinical question. For instance, if the question is abdominal pain, the answer should be placed concisely in this section. Always think of the impression as the answer to the reason for the study and your impressions will always be relevant and useful to the clinician ordering the study.

In addition, it is the most widely read part of the report. I like to say that the impression is for the clinician. The rest of the report is for the radiologist. In fact, many times the only part of the report that will be read by the referring doctor is the impression. So, make sure to spend the most time on this section. Check this part over many times to make sure what you are saying makes sense and is concise and relevant. Also, make sure to put your conclusions in this section of the dictation and anything that you think the physician will need to know such as management or follow-up.

Don't use technical jargon in this part of the report. The bane of the radiologist existence is getting phone calls for unimportant questions about technical terms within your dictation. It wastes lots of time and energy. I can assure you if you put terms in your report in this section that a clinician does not understand, you will get way too many unnecessary phone calls!!!

The impression should contain the most relevant conclusions in your dictation. So, for instance, if you describe the following in your comments section: *Within the liver, there is a hypervascular well-circumscribed mass in segment VI measuring 2.5 x 3.0 cm on image #51 with some peripheral nodular enhancement. Delayed imaging does not show typical centripetal filling. The differential includes most likely atypical hemangioma. Other etiologies such as a hepatic adenoma or hypervascular metastatic lesion are within the differential diagnosis but are less likely. MRI is recommended for further characterization.* Then the impression can say something like *Hypervascular segment VI hepatic mass. Consider most likely hepatic hemangioma. Correlate with abdominal MRI for further characterization.* If you notice, the most likely conclusion and the recommendation for further study is placed in the impression section. The other information can be left in the body of the report for further reading if necessary. This way the clinician knows what is most likely and what they should do next without the excess verbiage to potentially confuse the clinician.

What terms are most frowned upon in the impression?

Avoid the usage of *cannot be excluded.* This statement is usually unhelpful to the physician and does not provide any additional information to the reader. The sun can swallow the earth in the next hour. This cannot be excluded!!!! This statement will inflict the ire of the clinician and will lead to additional unnecessary workup because now the clinician has to a workup a very unlikely possibility. However, there is one condition for which I may use this term. In the setting of a positive pregnancy test and a negative pelvic ultrasound, I may say *ectopic pregnancy cannot be excluded* because I always want the clinician to follow the patient for an ectopic pregnancy with blood work/B-HCG levels regardless of the findings in my dictation. But that is the exception and not the rule!!!

Also, do not use the statement *clinical correlation is recommended*. Our job as radiologists is to correlate the radiological findings with the clinical findings. It is considered to be a lazy unhelpful statement in all situations. Don't make the radiologist look bad!!!

There are other terms that you will find that may irk some radiologists. Others may not care as much. I remember one attending who hated the use of the phrase *lung zone* and the use of the word *infiltrates* on a chest film. To this day, I do not use these phrases in my dictation because I do not think they are specific. However, I often come across these phrases in other radiologist's reports. So, you still need to abide by the quirks and specificities of individual radiology attendings. In the end, it is their name at the end of the report!!!

STRUCTURED REPORTING DICTATIONS VS. PROSE DICTATIONS

To start, structured reporting is basically a report itemizing the different findings in list form. Usually, it is organ based and may be a fill in the blank or a menu choice of items that the radiologist needs to pick. Using structured reporting vs. prose dictation styles is an area of controversy. Newly minted radiologists will more often apply the rules of structured reporting dictations and seasoned radiologists tend to use a more flexible prose style. But, there is a significant cross-pollination of both styles at all points in the career of radiologists. There is a great article from Radiology called <u>Structured Reporting: Patient Care Enhancement or Productivity Nightmare</u>. (1) I highly recommend you go to this URL if you are interested in learning the advantages and disadvantages of each style of dictation. However, I will summarize by saying that the key to a thorough and understandable dictation regardless of the style is to remember to adopt your own mental checklist and stick to the same program each time you make a dictation. You may adopt either style, as both can be appropriate.

Some departments, however, may have standardized dictations and may require the use of either of these styles. So, you need to abide by the rules of your department!

CONCLUSION:

Learning the basic mechanics of dictation is a rapid process. However, learning to dictate reports that are concise, relevant, and useful for the clinician takes the four years of residency and beyond to really hone your skills. I hope the guidelines above make your transition to a more professional dictation style a bit quicker and easier!

(1) http://pubs.rsna.org/doi/full/10.1148/radiol.2493080988

CHAPTER 11

What Clinicians Don't Want From A Radiologist- The 8 Deadly Sins

● ● ●

ONE OF MY READERS SENT me the following message, "I would really like you to write about what clinicians want from a radiologist." That comment initiated some thoughts about the topic since our primary goal as radiologists is to answer the clinician's questions. But, let's take this idea from a different angle. At some point in our careers, we all have made cardinal mistakes that really turn off our referring clinicians. What is more interesting than the mistakes that most of us have made at some point in our career to teach us lessons about how we can avoid angering our referring physicians and make things right for them? So, let's talk about what clinicians don't want from a radiologist! (The negative tends to be more interesting than the positive!) Let's give this a whirl...

THE FORCED HAND

In training and board examinations, we are often told to write recommendations for further management. So, how bad could it be to recommend a biopsy for a thyroid nodule when you see a new one? An angry head and neck surgeon stomps up to the department and looks for you. He yells loudly, "Why are you telling me what to do with my patient. He should not be getting a biopsy in this condition!!!" Bzzzzzzz... (Buzzer sound)

Pretty darn bad! When you write a recommendation, you have to remember that often times you don't have the full picture of the patient's situation. Or, in another word, there is asymmetry of information between the clinician, the radiologist, and the patient. Maybe, the patient can't lie flat. Perhaps, the patient can't handle needles. Possibly, there is an outside study only the clinician knows about. Or, there is some other issue that you can't imagine that the patient and the clinician are only privy to. By recommending a biopsy of a thyroid nodule without a caveat, for instance, you are legally forcing the clinician into having to investigate it further whereas it may not be the correct management protocol for the patient. I have learned to be very gentle with my management recommendations over the years!!! Always leave the clinician a way out...

INDECISIVENESS

We write a list of 10 items in our differential diagnosis without additional comment- like a laundry list in order to give a "complete differential". Days later you get a phone call from the clinician- "I don't understand what you are saying- what do you really think is going on here?"

How can we avoid this scenario? If you have a large differential diagnosis, always state what you think is most likely and why. Avoid delving too far into the 1 in a million diagnosis unless you have a real sneaking suspicion it might be the correct one. Clinicians appreciate when you make your best guess since it often will steer the doctor down the correct path. Too much information without direction can be bad!

THE SAUCY RADIOLOGY REPORT

You are angry that the referring physician did an inappropriate workup on a patient performing an iodine scan as a first test in a workup for a palpable thyroid nodule, whereas you know that it should be a thyroid ultrasound instead, so you put in your report the following statement, *Make sure to order the ultrasound instead of a thyroid scan in patients with palpable lump.* The doctor comes storming in, "How dare you to talk to me like this in your report. This is a legal document!"

If you have an issue with a clinician, make sure to air your dirty laundry outside of the report. The clinician is correct. You are putting the physician in a potential situation with legal liability. This sort of comment does not belong anywhere inside the report.

The Discrepant Report

You dictate a case from the night before when the overnight resident was on call. In the morning, you find a pulmonary embolus but you do not look at the additional documentation from the resident or the nighthawk. You do not call the doctors to let them know. Later in the day, the ER doctor walks up to the emergency department and says, "What the hell is going on here?" It turns out the overnight doctors did not call the study positive and sent the patient home. The physician was never notified...

Discrepant reports between you and other physicians can cause negligent patient care. Always make sure to check all the information to make sure that all parties are on the same page. Discrepancies will occur. But make sure to notify all parties!!!

Is It Better, Worse or Unchanged?

You are following a patient with breast cancer on a CT scan and you proudly discover and then mention a subtle liver lesion in your report. You refer to the prior study but don't really look at it. You also do not document the size of the lesions, nor compare the size of the lesions to the previous study. Two days later you get a phone call from the oncologist, "What is going with my patient? I need to know if I have to change chemotherapy. Are the hepatic masses changed?"

Clinicians always want to know if their patient is improving, unchanged, or has progressive disease. These imaging issues often change clinical management and are of the utmost importance to the clinicians. Always make sure to put these findings in the impression of your report!!!

INCOMPREHENSIBILITY

You look at a pelvic MRI on a patient with fibroids. The fibroids seem to be getting larger over time. However, you don't check over the report and click the sign off button. Before you know it, the report goes out to the clinician. Three days later you get a phone call from the doctor, "It says here in the body of the report that there is interval enlargement and in the impression, there is no interval enlargement of the fibroids. Which one is correct?"

Make sure to check for grammatical and logical statements within a completed dictation prior to signing it off. Very few things piss off a clinician more than not being able to understand what to do with their patient. An unclear report leads the clinicians down this pathway. Always check your report!!!

THE WRONG DIAGNOSIS

You are looking at a case of a patient with a type of arthritis that you have not seen for a while on a plain film. Finally, you decide to dictate the case without confirming the diagnosis via Google or running it by another clinician. You call it osteoarthritis. The patient gets treated based upon your report. One year later, the patient is still not getting better and the doctor sends a new film to another one of your colleagues. He comes up to you later in the day and states, "you dictated a case and called it osteoarthritis. It was a definite case of gout!!!"

If you are not sure about a diagnosis, always make sure to either look it up or run it by someone else. We are in the business of healing others. You should never have too much pride to make guesses when you can get the correct answer!!!

NOT ANSWERING THE CLINICAL QUESTION

You dictate a plain film of the chest and you happen to see a lytic lesion in the middle of the thoracic spine as well as a pulmonary nodule in the right lower lobe. So, you put in your impression- *MRI of the thoracic spine is recommended for further characterization. 8 mm right lower lobe pulmonary nodule.* A few days later you get a phone call from the physician- "We already know about the osseous lesion and it is a known hemangioma as seen in previous studies. The history said to compare the lung nodule with the prior study. Please take a look at that!"

It is imperative to scour the history for whatever clinical question the clinician wants to be answered. This way you can actually provide a helpful answer to improve patient care. That is the main reason we are here as radiologists!

The Eight Deadly Sins- Lessons Learned

As clinicians, we always need to self-reflect in order to improve our practice of medicine. There is no room for too much pride. We should constantly look for ways to improve our clinical skills, reports, and communications with our colleagues. I have just given you 8 different examples of issues that can arise if you want to cut corners. You can easily avoid further carnage to your own reputation, your patients' reputation, and your colleagues' reputation by remembering these situations. Use these examples as a template to avoid the eight deadly sins of a radiologist!

CHAPTER 12

Technology Essentials For the Radiology Resident (by Daniel Choe, D.O.)

● ● ●

IN AN ERA OF EXPONENTIAL technological growth, it is important that trainees use the latest technology to enhance their education. There is increasing demand upon the trainee to remain up to date and to have the ability to seamlessly access information. I venture to mention a few essential uses of technology that may help enhance the graduate training experience for the radiology resident. Different from many articles out there, I have no direct financial disclosures about the products I mention in this article.

SMART PHONE/TABLET

It seems like a no-brainer to have a smartphone/Ipad, but believe it or not, I once had a colleague who started residency with a blackberry. The Ipad or tablet may serve as a surrogate or mobile substitute for a laptop/notebook, but it has limitations in terms of storage and computational power. While upgrading them is easy due to its backup/sync features, it often lacks in ease of use for programs that require powerful graphics rendition or multi-program use. It is ideal for mobile use of editing online documents, viewing online lectures, storing a limited number of pdf files, and running apps for question banks. Several anatomy-learning apps are available and extremely useful for a fee. There is a separate section on apps later on.

CLOUD SERVICES

Most users already have cloud services. In fact, that is often the problem - there seem to be too many online storage services. Google, Amazon, Dropbox, OneDrive just to name a few. An elegant solution that helps consolidate all of the different clouds you may use is a service such as odrive. It is free, encrypted, and allows you to automatically sync when you copy files to the odrive folder on your computer. The caveat is that in order to use the sync feature you must have enough space on your hard drive. My suggestion is to invest in a cloud service that offers unlimited space and only the folders that you open most frequently. This is important for the resident who is constantly doing research and keeping tabs on what lectures and videos were watched. Or, if you use a pdf reader, it can keep track of which page you were on in one of many textbooks you will be inevitably reading.

COMPUTER

Regardless of whichever camp you fall into, Mac or PC, your home computer or laptop/notebook should be the workhorse for your education and work. I could write an entirely separate article, but for the sake of simplicity, I will say that a home desktop is not essential, but definitely a plus. Because cloud services work seamlessly and storage space is a problem of the past, your desktop is a great way to consolidate your work and use programs that require slightly higher computing power and graphics rendition. For example, I use a remote desktop to do a majority of my preparation for tumor board research, presentations, and research projects. I personally have my computer permanently connected to my flat screen TV as a secondary monitor so I can multitask. I am also able to watch lectures on my TV, which affords greater detail and definitely a plus when trying to take cases. I also recommend swapping out your primary hard drive for a solid-state drive (SSD) and adding a secondary storage drive. They are becoming more affordable these days. Keep in mind; much of the work can be accomplished with a laptop, MacBook, or even tablet/PC as well, at the cost of overall computational power and storage.

Universal Password Program

I use a password and personal information storage program, which over-all cuts out approximately 50 hours a year in retyping and resetting pass-words. I have over 200 passwords stored and am able to routinely change and generate new complex passwords in order to maintain security. It also allows you to store credit card information and secured notes for passwords and sensitive information. There are many services out there. I would select the one that suits your needs. It is definitely worth the money.

Remote Access

Most institutions provide remote access for its residents. If not, it behooves you to suggest that residents have access to remote PACS and EMR. This is critical not only for learning purposes but for effective workflow in prepa-ration for interdisciplinary rounds. Your time is better spent working or studying than having to schlep to the department or stay late (unless you are actively trying to avoid home for a particular reason).

Shared Network Storage

My institution did not initially provide shared in-network storage, but since its inception, we have been able to provide important resources for all residents and staff. More importantly, it serves as the institutional memory for a growing and developing residency program by eliminating the possibility of losing critical learning resources. It is also an excellent way to circumvent the elaborate HIPAA clauses in your IRB research protocol.

I will also include the necessity of a secured (password protected) USB drive as a conduit for transferring secure data between machines. Your program or IT department may provide one for you. If not, it will serve you well in the long run as it will allow you to transfer sensitive documents from your personal computer to a secured hospital network.

Apps

There are so many great apps available, but I can only mention a few that are essential for the resident. A document reader is critical. One that allows you to maintain a "bookmark" for each document you upload and open and save highlights and notes you want to review later. This is one that is worth a few dollars because it allows you to carry your library wherever you go, saves highlights directly onto the document, and saves your page position. I personally use <u>Goodereader</u> (1) for my Ipad, because it was one of the best at the time, but there may be new readers out there that suit your preferences.

Several of my colleagues purchased a group subscription for <u>e-anatomy</u>. (2) This app is a comprehensive anatomy atlas with corresponding radiology images.

<u>Radiology Assistant</u> (3) has recently developed a new app, which is an adaptation to its website. The app allows you to review all the content on their website while offline if the data is pre-downloaded. If you like the website as a resource, it is an even better tool as an app.

The different learning apps available can turn your phone into an instant tutor with quiz programs such as <u>Chegg</u> (4) or <u>Anki</u> (5) just to name a few. Also, most of the decks relevant to your training probably already exist. I found over 500 premade CORE exam cards. Use at your own risk since they cannot be vetted except throughout your own review. You can download and edit them as you go if you find the information is not up to date.

Conclusions

At the end of the day, your training experience relies heavily on how you learn. You may get by without some of the aforementioned technologies, so it's entirely up to you to decide what you really need. The items I have mentioned are recommended so that the resident, from day one, is able to optimize the use of time with relatively cheap resources (or otherwise covered/subsidized by your program). John Stuart Mill wrote, "there are many truths of which the full meaning cannot be realized until personal experience has brought it home." Hopefully, my experience will serve its purpose to jump-start your own journey through residency.

(1) http://goodereader.com

(2) https://www.imaios.com/en/e-Anatomy

(3) http://www.radiologyassistant.nl

(4) https://www.chegg.com

(5) https://apps.ankiweb.net

CHAPTER 13

How To Prepare For Interdisciplinary Conferences As A Radiology Resident

● ● ●

You get the email... There is a urology conference on Tuesday morning at 7 AM and you are responsible for showing 4 cases with multiple radiological studies. You've never done this before! How do you know which images to show? Is there a logical order to the images? Will I be able to answer the questions posed by the clinicians in the room? Your heart beats a bit faster as you contemplate the issues.

This situation is common for the beginning radiology resident. Often times, first-year radiology residents are thrust into their first interdisciplinary conference without much preparation. However, even though initially nerve racking as an experience, these conferences are a great opportunity to get to know your other medical colleagues as well as a way for them to find out about how knowledgeable you are!

Presenting for the interdisciplinary crowd is a bit different than preparing for the typical conference that you have been accustomed to over the years. Your audience is going to be a bit more sensitive to mistakes that are made by the presenter because decisions can often directly affect patient care. Therefore, I am going to discuss some of the common questions that arise when you encounter your first interdisciplinary conference to make you feel a bit more comfortable. These topics include how to sort through what is important, what to discuss, and when to ask for additional help in order to prepare for your first solo interdisciplinary conference as a radiology resident. So let's get started...

Selecting Cases

When going through a case, clinicians like to have the relevant initial diagnostic images and the subsequent follow-up images. So, it is imperative to get the correct history for the main diagnosis. When you check the computerized records, make sure to find all studies that support the main diagnosis. Then, you will need to look for the earliest studies of this sort. So, if the diagnosis is breast cancer, find the first mammogram and breast MRI that is present on the record. If the topic is metastatic colon cancer, look for the first CT scan showing the metastatic disease.

Next, you need to find the first post-treatment studies. So, find the next series of relevant studies. If the topic is a retroperitoneal bleed, find the first series post intervention cases such as the post-embolization CT scan. These will usually be the second from the beginning.

And, then finally, look for the most recent relevant studies. If this was that case of metastatic colon cancer, find the most recent CT scan of the abdomen and pelvis to show the final consequences of treatment or lack of treatment.

Selecting Individual Images

There are two ways to show images during a presentation. First of all, you can go to the source images in the PACS system and flip through the images directly. Or, you can select individual images and display them on a PowerPoint presentation. I would recommend doing the latter. Why? Simply, you leave less to interpretation by the audience. You will get a lot fewer questions regarding things that you are not sure about during the presentation and the clinician will less likely ask about information and findings that are irrelevant. For instance, you are less likely to get a question about that borderline enlarged node on the corner of the film that was not mentioned but is present on the PACS display. By choosing the PowerPoint format, you have much more control over what is displayed. This keeps the discussion centered on the important topics.

Also, there is less chance for technical issues. PACS systems have a tendency to go down when you most need it since it relies on an internet connection. A PowerPoint presentation is much more reliable since you do not have to rely upon the internet.

In addition, when choosing individual images make sure to look for the relevant information without the fluff. For instance, if it is that metastatic colon cancer patient, take those pictures only of the liver metastasis without the volume averaging artifact. If it is the retroperitoneal bleed, show only those images containing the bleed without other distracting findings on the film. And so on...

Discussions

When it is your turn to discuss a case, keep the discussion targeted. You want to only start discussing those issues that are relevant to the clinician's question. If they want to know if the metastatic colon cancer lesion is better, worse, or unchanged, provide the clinician the relevant information such as the measurements. If they want a differential diagnosis, provide it. But, do not go off on a tangential vector! If you go off topic, clinicians tend to get angry because of the limited time that you will have during the morning to discuss patient care and other cases. So, don't do it!

Also, try to look up relevant information on the topic during your preparations prior to participating in the conference. If you want to look like a star, gain additional knowledge on the relevant topics so that you can answer those questions intelligently and with authority. Then, you will establish an excellent reputation for yourself during the conference. Imagine how you will sound being able to describe the features of colon cancer metastasis if asked rather than muddling through and stuttering.

When To Ask For Help?

So, you've gathered your studies and selected your images. When is it appropriate to ask your attending for some assistance? Here are some specific circumstances: You have never rotated through a specific modality and you are presenting those images during that case. You are not sure that the report description is the same as the information on the images. You do not understand some of the disease entity issues that are going to be discussed.

Personally, I always like to know about any questions the resident may have prior to completing preparations for a conference. Better to be safe than sorry!!!

FINAL THOUGHTS

Preparing your first interdisciplinary conference can be a very stressful situation, especially if you do not have much basic guidance. Hopefully, this short summary will allow you to make more sense of the necessary preparations involved. Good luck with your next conference!

CHAPTER 14

Radiology Call- A Rite of Passage

● ● ●

EVERY YEAR AROUND THE BEGINNING of July, I see some of the most haunted radiology resident faces, right around 10:00 pm, just after the attending evening shift ends, and the resident night shift begins. It is almost always a second-year radiology resident who happens to be beginning his/her first night of call. What if I miss something important? What if I say something stupid? Will I be able to handle the intensity? Will I fall asleep? And most importantly, will I kill someone?

The answers to these burning questions are only unlocked after the resident takes the first night of call. It is only after this event that the resident and the program director know whether or not he/she can handle the burdens of a radiologist. Everything in the first year leads up to this point: the precall quiz, the intense reading, the conferences, and the studying. It's crunch time.

Just before the first night of dreaded call, my famous last words are: you begin the night as a boy/girl and you will end the night as a man/woman. Why do I say that? Because I think there is truth in that statement. Until you have the responsibility of independently making decisions for patients, you can never be a full-fledged radiologist. It's like all those ancient traditions in all religions/cultures like hunting that first wild boar, the confirmation, the bar mitzvah, etc. You are now allowed to function as an independent freethinking human being who can make decisions on your own. Until that point, you are merely an observer, not an active participant.

Since call is such an intense and important experience, there are multiple things you must do to make it valuable and safe. I am going to enumerate 8 simple golden rules of night call I wish I knew prior to beginning those fated first nights to come. I urge that all are followed in order to enrich your education in a safe manner. Do not stir the wrath of your fellow staff members and program directors in the morning by breaching these rules!

1. LOOK AT EVERY FILM WITH THESE PRIMARY THOUGHTS- WHAT WILL KILL THE PATIENT AND WHAT IS COMMON?

I can guarantee you that if you look at every film with these thoughts at the forefront of your brain and you have done the prerequisite work to get to call, you will not severely harm any of your patients. When you look at a chest film, always think pneumothorax. When you look at a female pelvic ultrasound, always think ruptured ectopic. When you look at a CT scan in a patient with right lower quadrant pain, always think acute appendicitis. And, so on, and so forth… Thinking about badness will prevent undiscovered horribleness in the morning.

Likewise, when you look at films always think about the most common diagnoses first and you will be right much more often than wrong. For instance: Opacity on a chest film- pneumonia, not Hampton's hump. Restricted diffusion on a brain MRI- infarct, not ependymoma. Abnormality on a GI bleeding scan, think primary GI bleed, not Meckel's diverticulum with bleeding gastric remnant. I can guarantee your attending will be looking at you funny if you come up with too many zebras!

2. ALWAYS, ALWAYS, ALWAYS MAINTAIN YOUR SEARCH PATTERN IN EVERY STUDY.

In the radiology world, one of the main ways to miss something is not to look for it. There are going to be times in the middle of the night when the pressure may seem insurmountable and you need to deliver an answer at that second. A team of 4 angry surgeons comes down and asks, "What is going on with the film?" and needs to know now! An inpatient resident shoves a chest film in front of your face and says, "What's going on here?" The emergency medicine doctor is calling incessantly to get a read on that CT chest for dissection. In each of these cases, I don't care how emergent and immediate they need the answer, always step back and go through your search pattern. This is a cardinal mistake that everyone makes at one time or another. Avoid it! Step back and say give me a moment. Go through each organ or region in a rigorous manner. You will look a hell of a lot less stupid than blurting a diagnosis/finding out only later to realize it was wrong because you haven't thoroughly analyzed the study. One of the worst feelings is having to find the doctor that just left your department with the wrong answer who is getting ready to begin surgery that is not needed or is going to discharge a patient that needs to stay in the hospital!!

3. If there is no harm to the patient, it is easier to do the study than to fight it.

This is one piece of sage advice that most residents take a while to learn. At nighttime, you will have limited time for everything. You are going to be pulled in fourteen different directions at once. You are going to be getting calls from the emergency department, the floors, the surgeons, etc. And often times, these events tend to happen all at once. So, I urge you that if there is a study that is reasonable, just do the study. You will spend more time and energy on preventing a study from getting done than just completing it. Of course, if the study is going to do significant harm to a patient, then obviously avoid it. But, that is the exception rather than the rule. That fluoroscopy study to rule out foreign body that you try to block after the resident ordered it: I can guarantee it will come back hours later when you are either exhausted or have lots of things going on at once. So, just do the study!!!

4. Don't let your temper get the best of you, you will hear about it in the morning!

There are going to be times for every resident when you encounter a curt gynecologist, a rude surgeon, a loud demanding resident, and so on. You yourself are likely going to be grouchy and tired as well. It may seem like a good idea to talk back to that person in a similarly rude and unprofessional manner. Or, you may want to take a swing at one of these annoying chaps. But, don't do it. One of the most common complaints we get at nighttime is a letter written by an attending or resident saying this radiology resident was unprofessional and handled the situation poorly under pressure. This will come regardless of whether the radiology resident is right or wrong. And often, it will stay in the resident's file/record. Don't let that be you!!!

5. Resident matters are best handled by residents. Attending matters are best handled by attendings.

At nighttime, there are going to be times when an attending radiologist is needed. Make sure you don't go in over your head. Call your attending when necessary. The worst thing that you can do in the morning is to perform a procedure that your attending should have done or make a phone call that really should have been handled by your attending, only to find out that the wrong thing happened. It will become the talk of the town among the department, and not in a good way... A brain scan always needs to be read by an attending because of litigation issues. An intussusception reduction should always be in the presence of a radiologist. And, so on and so forth... Don't go over your head!

Likewise, if there is a resident issue at nighttime, try to handle it yourself. If they are asking you whether to give the contrast or not, make that decision. If a resident comes down to ask a question, answer it. You will only learn how to make the smaller decisions by playing the role of a radiology resident.

6. ASK FOR HELP IF YOU CAN'T HANDLE SOMETHING AT NIGHTTIME.

There are going to be times when the job may be too much to bear for one person. (A disaster happened with every patient getting a full body CT scan) There are going to be questions that can only be answered by an expert. (A subtle abnormality on an emergent Neuro CTA) And, there are going to be administrative issues that can only be handled by your chairman or program director. (The MRI broke - should we recommend sending patients to another hospital?) If there are issues such as these that come up at nighttime, make sure to call the appropriate channels going from lowest to highest in command. If it is a patient question that you are not sure about, ask your chief resident. If he/she can't answer the question, you may want to ask the assigned attending on call. And, up the chain, it goes.

If you decide to handle everything yourself and it is inappropriate for your level, you can almost be certain that there will be repercussions in the morning. So please, ask for help when it is needed and appropriate!!

7. ALWAYS ANSWER YOUR BEEPER/PHONE/PAGER.

On occasion, we hear about a resident who was caught sleeping or not answering their pager at nighttime. Unfortunately, those residents will often get written up in the morning for lack of timely dictation, etc. So, simply jack up the sound on your beeper/phone/pager. And, take all calls!!!

8. LOOK AT THE FILMS. DON'T RELY ON THE ER OR NIGHTHAWK READS.

Being on call is the time to remove the umbilical cord and develop independence from your mentors/attendings. So, make sure not to repeat a dictation or reading that is already present. You should do everything de novo/from scratch although you should look at their reads afterward. It also looks really silly when the resident dictation matches the nighthawk dictation verbatim and hints that the resident may not have looked at the films. When I am on in the morning, I appreciate the extra set of eyes that a resident used to check the cases even though others have looked at the study. And, it is not infrequent that our residents catch important findings that the nighthawk didn't notice. So please, do your own independent reads/dictations!!!

SUMMARY STATEMENT

Call is a difficult but integral part of raising a radiology resident right. It is a time of trials and tribulations. You too can and will make it through this harrowing trial as you long as you follow the golden rules. Good luck!

CHAPTER 15

The Midnight Radiology Residency Discrepancy

● ● ●

IF YOU HAVEN'T HAD A discrepancy with the covering morning radiologist as a resident on call, you either haven't read enough cases, you are the long lost great great grandson of William Roentgen, or perhaps your name is Watson, the artificial intelligence computer, and you work for IBM!!! The truth that very few attendings seem to admit is that everyone, including attendings, will miss something every once in a while. In fact, one study reported radiologists clinically miss something important between 2-20% of the time. (1) From my experience, that number seems very high, but nonetheless, the rate is significant enough. So, when... and notice, I don't say if... you miss something and have a discrepancy at nighttime, you are actually being a normal radiology resident. I would even go as far to say that you are actually fortunate, in a sense, because you didn't miss the finding as a full-fledged attending. You have someone to back you up and hopefully, you will never miss that finding again.

The first step, of course, is to prevent the major misses. The cases you need to study leading up to taking call are the cases that are common and lead to significant morbidity and mortality. You want to literally view hundreds of different types of appendicitis, aortic ruptures, pulmonary emboli, and so on and so forth so that when the time comes for you to take call, the chance of missing the important finding is significantly decreased. Unfortunately, however, we can't prevent all the inevitable misses, and frankly, we have to admit it to ourselves first and foremost that this will be the case.

So, what do you do when you have a significant miss? Maybe you sent a patient home with acute appendicitis or a patient with a ruptured ectopic pregnancy. Maybe you missed an early retroperitoneal bleed. In any of these cases, there are certain keys to making the discrepancy, not just another horrible encounter, but rather a learning experience that is valuable for the remainder of your career. We will go a through a few rules that you need to follow in the rest of this chapter.

DON'T PERSEVERATE

The first important point is how you emotionally react to the discrepancy. It is also a life lesson. We can't undo what is done. You need to move on... Perseverating about a miss is counterproductive at best and can cause future misses at worst. Remember, just because you made a significant miss does not mean you are or will be a horrible radiologist. So, you need to get over it. The same rules apply to questions on written exams, future failures, etc. One miss does not a radiologist make...

MAKE SURE TO FOLLOW-UP THE PATIENT IN THE MORNING

When you find out about the bad news, it is bad form just to leave the department sulking, not attempting to make good on the miss that you made. Try to do what you can to make sure that the physicians in the emergency room know there was a discrepancy. Or, you may need to call the patient back yourself, if need be. Bottom line... You need to make an effort to clean up your mess. It is partially your responsibility.

READ ALL YOU CAN ABOUT THE MISS TO NOT MAKE THE MISTAKE AGAIN

Reading about the case; reviewing the films; looking at other similar cases: These are all the things you should be doing soon after the miss. This is a real opportunity to understand and fix the incomplete knowledge you had on the subject before, and, of course, to never make the same mistake again.

Teach Others

One of the most rewarding ways of compensating for the discrepancy is to make your fellow residents and junior residents aware of the miss. Teaching your colleagues protects them from making the same mistake that you have made. And, even better, it reinforces the knowledge you have, thereby making it much less likely that you will repeat the same mistake. Just like lightening, it rarely strikes twice!!!

Final Thoughts

Midnight discrepancies are part of the normal learning ritual for a radiology resident. It is not the discrepancy itself that is a problem. That is to be expected and is part of the normal routine residency learning experience. But rather, the issue is how you as a radiology resident learn and grow from the experience. Make the best of a tough situation!!!

(1) https://www.ncbi.nlm.nih.gov/pmc/articles/PMC3609674/ Discrepancy and Error in Radiology: Concepts, Causes, and Consequences

CHAPTER 16

How Far Should I Take That Procedure?

● ● ●

THE SITUATION

YOUR RADIOLOGY ATTENDING TELLS YOU to interview a patient and then complete an ultrasound guided breast biopsy, knowing that it was a large mass and a fairly simple case. You have done this procedure numerous times with this same attending. So, you go ahead and do it again. No complications. No issues. When you are done with the procedure, you feel immense pride in your capabilities. You show the attending the pictures from the biopsy. The attending congratulates you on a job well done.

Round 2 later that same day.... A different radiology attending wants you to work up a different patient and start the next breast biopsy. So, you begin to interview the patient, set up the table and the sterile field, position the patient for the procedure, and place the ultrasound probe on the site of the biopsy. You begin to numb the overlying skin with lidocaine and make a small incision for the biopsy gun. Since the attending still has not shown up, you decide to place the needle right near the lesion, hit the targeted breast nodule and then subsequently collect multiple samples, placing each one into a little sterile cup on the side to be sent to pathology. You complete the rest of the procedure without complication. All seems to be well.

You clean up everything and let the patient know that everything went just fine. And, you tell her you are going to consult with the attending before you have her leave. So, you merrily step out of the room and walk down the hallway toward the radiologist's office to let her know about the patient's biopsy you completed. You enter the office and state, "I completed the biopsy successfully on patient "XYZ". The attending stares at you with a stern angry face and says "How dare you complete the procedure without consulting with me!!!" You are the talk of the department for the next month!

Unfortunately, during radiology residency, you may encounter similar situations such as this one. Different attendings have entirely varying expectations for radiology residents. Some may expect you to start and finish all procedures. Others may be less likely to allow the resident to have independence, even though he/she may be very capable. So what to do? I am going to go through several guidelines in assessing whether you, as a radiology resident, should complete a given procedure on your own.

Are You Competent In The Procedure?

This should be the first question that you need to ask as a radiology resident. If you do not think you have done enough of a procedure independently from start to finish, you certainly have no business doing any procedure or a portion of a procedure alone. Comfort level is also just as important. Even if you have the numbers of procedures behind you, if you do not feel comfortable with a procedure, you should also continue to make sure that you have your attending's guidance at all times until you have the comfort level that you need.

Are We Doing the Procedure For The Right Reasons?

Prior to performing any procedure, interventional or otherwise, you need to make sure that it has some clinical benefit. Nurses regularly come up to me and ask, "Should we give intravenous contrast?" The first thing I ask them in response is, "Why are we doing the study?" It may not need contrast in the first place. Likewise, no matter how inconsequential a procedure is, you always need to think about if it is necessary first!!!

Level of Difficulty of Procedure/ Potential For Complications

Some procedures such as a fluoroscopic upper GI series have a much lower complication rate than a complex oncological liver embolization. So, it is important to assess the difficulty and potential complications of any given procedure before deciding whether you should tackle it on you own. Most liver embolizations, stent placements, and angioplasties should probably be under the direct supervision of an attending unless perhaps you are about to graduate from an interventional fellowship in a few days. On the other hand, a paracentesis, although with the potential for some complications, can certainly be performed from start to finish by a resident.

Attending Expectations

Some attendings expect the resident to do almost everything and others feel the need to hold the resident's hand at every step. Much of that decision may be related to the trust between the attending and resident. However, it is extremely important to listen to the guidance of your attending prior to beginning or ending any procedure. Because you are not the physician that signs off on everything, you really need to abide by the rules of the person that is in charge. Always make sure to get the OK from the supervising physician prior to performing **any** procedure!

Patient Expectations

Many patients have an expectation for an attending to complete a procedure. Always abide by the wishes of the patient. You never want to be caught in a situation where the patient does not want you to be performing a procedure and you do so anyway. This is the realm of lawsuits and legal issues!!!

Summary Statement

The difficulty of residency can be more about self-assessment/awareness and working with colleagues than it is about the actual day-to-day mechanics of performing cases. You as a resident, need to always be aware of your own strengths and weaknesses as well as your expectations. My advice: make sure to always know in advance that you are performing a procedure for the right reasons, have the abilities to perform any procedures, and are expected to complete a procedure. Only then should you consider doing a procedure independently.

CHAPTER 17

Taking Oral Radiology Cases- A Lost Art?

● ● ●

THE LIGHTS GO DOWN AS the radiology attending in the front of the class-room prepares the computer for a case presentation. A switch is flicked on and a black and white PowerPoint case suddenly begins to shine brightly on the screen in front of you. The radiologist glances about the room looking to see who would be the best fit for this next case. You begin to sweat and fidget with your hands, praying that you will not be called on next. Suddenly the attending's glance remains fixed upon you. He says "Tell me about this patient with a 2-year history of a cough!" You become flustered and are not sure what to say.

The scenario above is a common daily occurrence in radiology resi-dencies across the country. However, over the past few years, I have noticed an overall decrease in proficiency in the way that residents present each radiological case. The art has been partially lost. Some of it may be related to poor teaching on our part. Some of it may be related to decreas-ing time allotted to teaching. Some of it may be related to the emphasis of the new board examination system. And, perhaps some may be related to changes in newer radiology resident class culture. In whatever case, it is a shame. Taking cases orally is a crucial step to becoming a well-rounded radiologist. You need to be able to convey to your colleagues' important information about the images in a timely logical manner, no matter what you are looking at. If you want to look like a star, you need to have this process down cold. So, in order to enable you to have the tools to get through a radiological case, I am going to go through the basics including determining the kind of study, presenting descriptive findings, coming up with a differential diagnosis, and ultimately determining proper management.

What The Bleep Am I Looking At?

Whenever you are introduced to a new case, the first thing you need to do is determine what you are looking at. Take your time and think about what kind of images you are shown. Many times the case discussion is lost even before it is begun because the correct study is never identified. Is it an ultrasound, CT scan, MRI, x-ray, or nuclear medicine study? Is the examination performed with or without contrast? During what phase is it?

For nuclear medicine studies in particular, if you can identify what the study is prior to beginning to go through the rest of the case, 80 percent of the heavy lifting has already been done. You have already isolated the differential diagnosis if you can identify the radiopharmaceutical. So, if you are not sure, you should start describing the physiological distribution of activity that is present to help with identification. Often times the act of describing the distribution, helps the resident to understand the type of study.

Also, scan the images for any identifying information. If it is an ultrasound, it will often tell you which organ you are looking at. I have found it can often be difficult to tell the testes, ovaries, and kidneys apart on a single image if it is not labeled. Usually, these studies are labeled so you will be able to differentiate among the options.

Finally, make sure to look at the top of the film to see if you can find the patient's age and sex. This can also further help you to hone in upon the correct differential diagnosis.

Describing The Findings

It is this part of the oral case when the newer residents fall short compared to residents that have studied to take the oral boards. Residents have a tendency to stop very quickly at the description part of the puzzle and then enter rapidly into a differential diagnosis. A poor quick description often times leads to a poor differential diagnosis. Again, you need to take your time to describe all the salient points.

So, what should be included in this part of the case? Always make sure to describe the location, the size, the intensity (if nuclear medicine), the shape, the density, and borders. Describe its effect upon adjacent structures. Make sure to use buzzwords if available. If it is an angry looking mass on CT scan that looks like a star, you may want to use the words spiculated or stellate. If it is a lesion with enhancing rim nodularity that fills in from the edge to the center, use the terms peripheral nodular enhancement with centripetal filling. These buzz words connote certain types of differentials in the minds of the radiologist listeners that provide information on the type of disease entity even prior to going through a differential diagnosis.

Finally, don't get happy eye syndrome. Look for other findings that may support or refute your differential diagnosis. I can't tell you how many times a resident will stare at one section of the film only to forget to look at the rest of the images or the rest of the film, and lose the forest for the trees.

Concise Relevant Differential Diagnoses

The difference between a novice and a more seasoned resident is stark when it comes to giving a concise and relevant differential diagnosis. The novice will either have no idea what to say or will continue to drone on about multiple different possibilities for the final diagnosis. They do not even differentiate between the zebra and the most common diagnosis.

Again, take your time before speaking. Prior to even starting this process, in your own mind, you should be going through broad categories of what the differential should be. Is it neoplasm, infection, inflammation, iatrogenic, congenital, etc.? Then, when you have come up mentally with some reasonable possibilities make sure to talk about no more than 3 etiologies of what are the most likely diagnoses. And, start with the most likely and then go down in order to the least likely. This process will allow you to speak logically as well as show that you have really thought about the differential in an analytical manner.

What Next For The Patient?

There are really three options for the further management of the case after you have completed the basics of determining the findings and differential diagnosis. The first possibility: no further workup is needed and a final diagnosis has been established. One example would be an adrenal nodule with a Hounsfield unit of 2. This finding would be consistent with an adrenal adenoma. End of story. No further workup needed.

Alternatively, it may be imperative that another step needs to be further worked up immediately. For instance, if you need to determine the matrix of an aggressive osseous lesion on a musculoskeletal MRI without a final diagnosis, make sure to recommend a plain film. Otherwise, the final disposition of the patient may never be determined.

And lastly, there may be a lesion that has low clinical significance but needs to be followed over time. In this category would be the small lung nodule or the nonaggressive indeterminate liver lesion.

You can almost always categorize your case into one of these three groups. And, it will show that you really thought about the ramifications of the imaging upon the clinical picture of the patient.

Final Thoughts: Taking Oral Cases Should Be Fun!!

Taking imaging cases orally should not be a difficult or embarrassing process. In fact, it should become something that you should look forward to in order to build your confidence and make you into a better radiologist. It is a summation of the most important ingredients needed to make an excellent radiologist: the ability to make the findings, synthesize the data, come up with an outcome, and communicate the results to the clinician.

Unfortunately, at many programs, you are just expected to know how to take a case without having been taught the process. If that is the case, at least now, you have a framework of the basic fundamentals of how to take a case outlined above. Just like anything else, being adept at taking cases orally, is simply a matter of practice and knowing the process. Once you have the process down and the base knowledge, it is much easier to build upon your abilities and become better and better over time. You too can become a star at taking cases!!!

CHAPTER 18

Tackling Research- Basic Issues And Considerations For The Radiology Resident

● ● ●

PUT AN ACADEMIC RADIOLOGIST AND a general community radiologist in the same room and start a conversation on research and radiology residency. How do you think that conversation would go? I bet there would be bitter debate and sharp words (kind of like the recent Clinton/Trump run for the presidency!). In fact, it would likely be next to impossible to get them both to agree on the merits of radiology research.

The academic radiologist would point out the necessity of research to allow the resident to understand how to delve deeply into an area within radiology, really understand the mechanics of how discoveries are made, and to create and advance new areas of knowledge within our specialty. He would espouse the importance of statistically analyzing false positive and negative rates, ROC curves, sensitivities, and specificities, tools that are invaluable to becoming a good radiologist. Additionally, he/she would also likely say that without an understanding of the mechanics of the research process, you can easily be misled by marketing and headlines for new software, contrast agents, radiology hardware, etc. that may at best marginally displaying the truth of an imaging process or at worst can be entirely incorrect.

On the other hand, the community radiologist would say that if you understand the fundamentals, can read films well, and know how to manage patients appropriately then what is the point of doing research? Let others come up with new ways of interpreting films, creating protocols, or creating new contrast agents. Or in other words, "leave the research to the academics". The community radiologist would also utter in the same breath that research is too time-consuming and costly as well as incompatible with the day to day running of a revenue generating practice. Why bother?

So, given these diametrically opposite points of view, the big question becomes: to what extent should the radiology resident pursue research during residency? Should you make it into an all-consuming process or should you relegate research to just satisfying the requirements of your residency program? Given the potential difficulties of making this decision for some residents, I am going to go through how to figure out for yourself whether you should follow the advice of the academic or community radiologist. In addition, if you go down the research pathway, I am going to give some sage advice about how to find a research mentor and what makes the best research projects.

How Much Research Should I Pursue?

Ever read about <u>Maslow's Hierarchy of Needs</u>? (1) If not, I highly recommend you click on the previous Wikipedia link. Instead of the Maslow's Hierarchy of Needs, now picture the Radiology Residency Hierarchy of Needs. At the base perhaps you would have reading lots of films, studying, and lectures. At the apex, you would have radiology research. The reason why this point is so important: your own basic needs of a radiology residency must be satisfied before you really can tackle the research requirement. Therefore, some questions that you must answer prior to tackling a research project would be: Have you been studying enough, attending lectures, and learning the basics of radiology concepts? Are you performing well on your rotations? Do you have to concentrate on other issues such as the USMLE? In other words, the resident needs to first focus on becoming a good radiologist and then his/her research. Without the essential elements of a good radiology residency preparation, the entire pyramid will collapse. Why do I make this statement? If the resident is concentrating so heavily on research instead of learning all the imaging modalities and vital skills during his/her residency program, he/she will find it very difficult to perform well during residency. You want to make sure that you know the general skills of the radiologist first and foremost. Furthermore, too much emphasis on research can potentially lead the resident to lose focus on other issues such as passing the core examination. So, make sure not to forget about the main reasons that you are doing your residency: to become a radiologist.

On the other hand, if you are able to dedicate time to research because you are comfortably able to divide your time appropriately, by all means, go for it. The rewards are numerous from both a practical as well as an academic standpoint. If you are interested in academic radiology, love to come up with innovative ideas, and enjoy writing publications then significant research becomes very important. Publishing several papers and abstracts during residency and fellowship can really help to get that first job if you are interested in pursuing an academic career.

Even in private practice, performing research during your residency shows that you take an interest in radiology. From a community radiology job market perspective (although the community radiologist may not want to admit it!), if you have two equal candidates, one who has accomplished much research and the other that has done none, I believe that most practices would choose to hire the former.

The bottom line- yes, research can be rewarding but make sure that it doesn't interfere with your basic mission of becoming a radiologist!

How Do I Find A Research Mentor?

Most radiology programs have some attendings that are almost exclusively clinical and others that are more academic. I would recommend that you seek out those mentors/attending that have a decent amount of research experience. Although these clinically based attendings can be great teachers and mentors for learning radiology, they will likely not be as useful for the pursuit of really understanding how to do research. In fact, although they may express interest in helping you out with research, often times, they will not be able to instruct you with how to complete a project. So, unless you already have a lot of experience with radiology research, a more clinically based radiologist may not be the best choice for a radiology research mentor. There are a lot of radiology attendings out there that don't really have a clue how to structure a research project. (Not that it makes them bad radiologists!)

Although it is not always possible depending on the size and structure of your residency program, also try to find a mentor in an area/subspecialty of radiology that interests you. He/she is more likely to help you out in your career since you have similar interests.

Finally, try to find a mentor that meshes with your personality. In addition to the grunt work of research, part of the research process involves bouncing ideas off one another and brainstorming. If you feel you are not an equal participant in the process, interesting research can begin to seem more of a chore than a true passion. It shouldn't be that way. Personality can become a significant issue.

What Makes The Best Research Projects?

My favorite research projects are those issues and problems that have constantly nagged at me or annoyed me over the years of practice that you have a hankering to solve. In addition, I love research projects that are in an area of true interest. These tend to be the best and most satisfying projects. I find that esoteric projects without real relevance do not really provide that spark to take the research to the next level. It also may dissuade the resident from pursuing other projects down the line.

I recommend that when you are involved in day-to-day readouts try to take notice of the issues that bother the attendings or questions that occur in the areas of interest that you really love. There are few things more satisfying than coming up with a question that you thought about and then figuring out how to solve it.

Final Thoughts

Radiology research is an excellent avenue for understanding the mechanics of what we do as radiologists. We rely upon many presumed facts for granted, whereas these facts may not be based on the best evidence available. Performing your own projects really allows the radiology resident to understand how to determine what information are true facts and what information does not have a basis in science. This process thereby helps the resident to read and interpret studies, and critically determine the accuracy of the information we use to interpret images on a day-to-day basis.

Furthermore, delving into research by completing a project can be a very satisfying professional endeavor as well as can become a capstone on top of your radiology residency training. In fact, I find there are few things more satisfying than answering your own question to which the body of literature did not provide an answer.

However, it is important to remember, you as a radiology resident, need to satisfy the basic needs of radiology residency first and foremost. Before making a final decision on whether or not to become involved in a project, consider if you really have the time and energy to pursue the project to its end. If a research project is very involved and time-consuming, think twice about the project because your first priority should be to become a well-trained radiologist. Radiology research can be rewarding, but only to the extent that you are first satisfying the basic requirements of radiology residency training.

(1) https://en.wikipedia.org/wiki/Maslow's_hierarchy_of_needs

CHAPTER 19

Book Reviews For The Radiology Core Examination (by Daniel Nahl, M.D.)

● ● ●

STUDYING FOR THE ABR CORE Exam is undoubtedly a daunting task. Not only can the sheer amount of material one needs to learn seem overwhelming, but also the vast amount of resources available can be more of a burden than an asset. I often see my fellow residents scrambling to make time to go over every single review book out there, in an effort to have all of their bases covered. This strategy is not only nearly impossible but is likely counterproductive. Rather, one should focus on one "comprehensive" review book while supplementing with case review books and question banks that work best for them.

When asking my peers about their thoughts on different study resources, I could never get a good consensus on what was best. Different people had the same success passing the exam with very different approaches. However, one commonality I did notice amongst those who had success on the exam was that their approach was comprehensive (covered all categories tested) and diligent. With that being said, it is best to first peruse a resource to make sure it is useful for your style of learning before fully committing your time (and money) to it. Also, it should be noted that none of these are substitutes for a comprehensive textbook (such as Brant and Helms or the Requisites series). Review books are most effective when they are, in fact, used as a review and not a primary source of learning.

Below are reviews of the resources my colleagues and I used, some more than others, to prepare for the ABR Core Exam.

COMPREHENSIVE REVIEW BOOKS
CORE RADIOLOGY: A VISUAL APPROACH TO DIAGNOSTIC IMAGING

This is an excellent review book that can be used as a single source for reference and overview of salient points. It contains lots of good quality images and diagrams (in color!), as well as tables summarizing differential diagnoses with easy ways to differentiate one entity from another. As with any review book, it may not delve into as much depth in any single topic. Supplementation with Brant and Helms, StatDX, or Radiographics articles may be required for certain topics that require more depth or clarity. This book can be easily understood by junior residents throughout their first or second years of residency, not simply just for those reviewing for the Core Exam.

One drawback of this textbook is its size. At 895 pages, it can be a pain to lug around. Also, compared to Crack the Core, this text lacks humor and motivational quotes. Rather it's more of a traditional, no-nonsense, and well-organized review.

CRACK THE CORE

Written under a pen name by "Prometheus Lionhart," this series includes two main volumes, together encompassing the main sections covered on the Core Exam. In addition to the main two-volume set, Lionhart has also written a separate dedicated physics review book as well as a case review book (which I will cover separately). This two-volume set is another excellent review source. While it covers much of the same material as Core Radiology, this text is geared specifically for passing the Core Exam by incorporating test-taking strategies in addition to providing factual information. Lionhart interjects jokes and motivational phrases to keep the reader entertained while studying (not an easy task!). This book is much more simplified than <u>Core Radiology</u> but serves as an excellent review for someone with solid background knowledge of the topics included. The physics and non-interpretive skills chapters in <u>Crack the Core</u> are much more robust and comprehensive than in <u>Core Radiology</u>. Additionally, Lionheart has a video lecture series to supplement his books (at an additional cost, of course), which can be useful depending on your style of learning.

One of the main drawbacks of the <u>Crack the Core</u> series is the abundance of typos in the text. While the typos generally don't alter the context, they can be an annoyance. Another downfall of <u>Crack the Core</u> is the image quality and lack of color diagrams. The supplementary video lecture series does have improved image quality and nice color diagrams and animations, however.

● ● ●

CASE REVIEW BOOKS
<u>CORE REVIEW SERIES</u> (THORACIC, GU, GI, MSK, BREAST, CARDIAC, NUCLEAR MEDICINE)

The newest of the main case review books, the Core Review Series has separate books in <u>Thoracic</u>, <u>Genitourinary</u>, <u>Gastrointestinal</u>, <u>Musculoskeletal</u>, <u>Breast</u>, <u>Cardiac</u>, and <u>Nuclear Medicine</u>. Each book is broken down into chapters, with each chapter covering a specific subcategory (usually starting out with fundamentals of imaging for that category or normal anatomy).

The good: The breakdown by chapter and multiple questions per chapter allows you to hone down your studying to a specific topic and to do multiple questions in a relatively short time period. Image quality varies by book but is generally very good. Most books have online access with an easy interface for doing questions (almost feels like a Q bank).

The descriptions for the answers are excellent. I feel that these books best prepare you to think the way they want you to think during the test; to understand the process of why an answer is right rather than regurgitate memorized information. Many of the books even have physics concepts integrated into the questions, which is a tactic the ABR often employs on the Core Exam.

The bad: When using the physical books, it can be tedious to flip between the questions and the answers (which are located at the end of the chapter). This problem is alleviated with the online versions, where the answers are available immediately after taking the question. Also, because not all subjects are covered, other sources must be used to supplement these areas (such as Interventional, Neuro, and Pediatrics).

RAD CASES (CARDIAC, GI, GU, INTERVENTIONAL, MSK, NEURO, NUCLEAR MEDICINE, PEDIATRICS, THORACIC)

Rad Cases offers a case-based approach (rather than the more question/answer format of Core Review Series) with approximately 100 cases per book. Each case shows images and a clinical presentation on the first page. The next page then goes over the imaging findings, differential diagnosis (with brief descriptions of each diagnosis and how it may or may not explain the imaging findings), essential facts about the disease entity, other possible imaging findings, and finally pearls & pitfalls.

The good: This series really does a good job of allowing the reader to come up with a systematic approach to a case. The explanations do a good job of highlighting how one may have fallen into a trap or how one should tailor their thought process when approaching a case. All of these are essential aspects of passing the exam.

The bad: While learning how to approach an unknown case is necessary to tackling exam questions, this text appears more driven to prepare residents for the old oral boards. One could argue that a more rapid-fire question/answer format is more useful when it comes to preparation for the Core Exam.

Case Review Series (Neuro, Head and Neck, Spine, Breast, Cardiac, Emergency Medicine, GI, GU, MSK, Nuclear Medicine, Pediatrics, Thoracic, Interventional)

Case Review Series (CRS) is another case based review, with each book separated into three different difficulty levels. The cases at the beginning of the book, "Opening Round," are easiest, the next level of difficulty in the middle of the book is termed "Fair Game" and the most difficult cases at the end are in the "Challenge" section. Each case shows images and is followed by four questions pertaining to those images.

The good: The book offers excellent cases with good image quality. The multiple questions per case really force you to learn several aspects about a case. When it comes to the Core Exam, knowing the diagnosis alone usually does not suffice. Thus, being able to answer questions from several angles about a case is a valuable learning tool.

The bad: Similar to Rad Cases, CRS appears to be more driven toward oral board prep. While this may help with expanding one's knowledge base, it lacks the multiple-choice question/answer that is necessary for the Core Exam. Also, the Challenge sections are often too difficult/esoteric and are often beyond the scope of the exam. It would behoove you to do only the Opening Round and Fair Game sections in order to save precious study time.

● ● ●

Physics/Other
Huda's Review of Radiologic Physics

This is the physics review book by Walter Huda, who administers yearly review courses in radiologic physics throughout the country. It is in bullet point form and aligns closely with his course.

The good: The book has pretty much everything you need to know for physics for the Core Exam, with review questions at the end of each chapter and online access. It is formatted in bullet point form to be intended for quick review. I used this book while at Huda's review course and immediately after it in order to reinforce the concepts he taught.

The bad: While all the facts you need to know may be in this book, there is very little in the way of explanation. You will have to use other, more thorough sources for a deeper understanding. Also, the questions at the end of the chapter serve to reinforce some basic topics but are unlike anything you will see on the exam.

Radiologic Physics "War Machine" by Prometheus Lionhart

This is the dedicated physics book by the Crack the Core author, with a very similar layout to Crack the Core.

The good: This book was a great resource for studying physics. It really simplifies topics and makes them easier to understand, and therefore memorize. He does a good job of explaining what physics is relevant to the test and what is not, which is extremely valuable (the last thing we want to do is study more physics than we need to).

The bad: Again, the typos. Also, there is a lot of overlap between this book and the physics section of the Crack the Core book. I have not examined them in detail, but I just studied the section in Crack the Core without using the War Machine book and felt it was more than adequate preparation.

● ● ●

Question Banks
RADPrimer

RADPrimer is the question bank associated with StatDx and has an abundance of questions (2,221 Basic and 3,747 Intermediate level questions).

The good: Lots of questions with mostly very good explanations. Good image quality. What I found most useful about RADPrimer was the ability to hone down the focus to exactly what I wanted to study. For example, if I had just read a section in a review book about CNS Infections,

I could create an exam and do those specific questions in order to solidify what I had just read.

The bad: Many of the questions are too straightforward for what you will see on the test. Rather it should be used as a learning tool to reinforce recently studied material and not a means to simulate the Core Exam. Also, while there are some physics questions, there are not enough to use these as the sole source of physics practice.

BoardVitals

BoardVitals is an online question bank that offers subscriptions based on different time increments ($399 for six months, $229 for three months, $139 for one month). There are 1500 questions broken up by general category.

The good: The questions better simulate the real exam than RADPrimer. The explanations on most questions are good. There are more physics questions than on RADPrimer and this bank also includes non-interpretive skills questions (which I found very helpful). What I also found very helpful was that the interface was well suited for use on mobile devices. Whether I was in a line somewhere, on a train, or on a bus I could bang out a few BoardVitals questions with ease.

The bad: Some of the answer explanations were one line without much information. These inadequate explanations happened once in a while and could be frustrating at times.

Face the Core

Face the Core is another online question bank, with 35 different modules. Each module has about 75-100 multiple-choice questions. Modules consist of several cases, with each case having approximately 4-5 associated questions. Modules can be purchased individually for $10 each or you can purchase all 35 modules for $250. Modules must be completed in full (all 75-100 questions) before you could go over the answers (no "tutorial" mode).

The good: I used this question bank at the end, to brush up on my weaker areas, so I liked that I could purchase just the modules I needed rather than forking over $250. The explanations were pretty good. Some of the modules even had video explanations, which was nice because they would go into more detail. The physics modules on Physics Artifacts and MRI Sequences were very helpful.

The bad: The main drawback is that you have to do the entire module before you can go over the questions. This made the process very time-consuming (at least 2 hours per module). The image quality was poor and the layout appeared somewhat haphazard. Overall it is a good resource to use at the end, to cover areas of weakness.

● ● ●

I know it seems daunting with all the resources out there. Don't be afraid to use many, but use them wisely. Below is a rough plan of how I approached studying for the exam. And it worked for me:

My approach:

6-8 months before the test

- Used **Core Radiology** early and often as primary source
- **RADPrimer** questions (based on exactly what I was studying in Core Radiology)

4-6 months before the test

- Continued above
- Started **Crack the Core Physics** (supplemented by various YouTube videos)
- Started **BoardVitals** Questions
- **Core Review Books**

2-4 months before

* Continued above (but started phasing out RADPrimer)
* **RadCases** and **Case Review Series** to supplement weak areas

1-2 months before

* Skimmed **Crack the Core** to fill any gaps/get different perspective
* Continued **BoardVitals**
* Started **Face the Core** on weak areas

≤ 1 month

* Crammed facts
* Reviewed notes
* Questions, questions, questions

Good luck!!!!

CHAPTER 20

The Chief Radiology Resident- An Insider's Perspective

● ● ●

EVERY YEAR AROUND THE DEAD of winter in our program, the program directors sit around a table and discuss who is going to be the next year's chief resident. Some years the decision is so easy that it takes no more than a few minutes. Other years the discussion is extremely cumbersome and may slog on over days or weeks. Some years everyone is happy with the decision. Other years no one is happy with the decision. Some years the chief resident role seems like a natural fit. Other years it is a role that we cannot imagine anyone could fill. Some years everyone wants it. Other years no one wants it.

It may seem like a mystery box to many of you why we have a chief resident, what exactly he/she does, and how this decision is made. So, this is a perfect opportunity to enlighten the audience. Today I am going to talk about the roles of a chief resident, the perks and downsides of the job, the issues that can make the decision to be a chief radiology resident easy or difficult, and how the choice is finally made.

WHAT IS THE ROLE OF A CHIEF RADIOLOGY RESIDENT?

Roles and responsibilities may vary slightly from program to program across the country. But the essence of a chief radiology resident usually remains the same. The chief resident is the liaison between the resident program and the program directors/attendings. Issues that arise with the residents are often brought first to the chief resident and then to the program director or responsible attending. Likewise, issues that arise from the attendings that affect the residents are often brought to the attention of the chief resident first, who then disseminates the information to the residents.

The duties of a radiology resident can include but are not limited to administrative scheduling of residents, scheduling noon conferences, scheduling board reviews, running review courses for medical students and junior residents, voting as a member of the educational committee, attending chief resident conferences such as the **AUR meeting** (1), scheduling guest lecturers, planning budgetary arrangements for the residency, interviewing medical students, and more. The responsibilities are great and the chief resident needs to command the respect of both the attendings and residents alike.

Downsides and Benefits

Just like any role with important responsibilities, there are significant ups and downs to being the chief resident. Let's start with the downside. From my experience, the chief resident is often held responsible for conflicts that can occur among the residents and between the attendings and residents. In fact, they tend to be caught in the middle of many of these issues. Often times, there are no perfect outcomes. In addition, the role of the chief resident can be time-consuming and challenging. The scheduling of residents alone is often fraught with lots of emotion and charged conflicts. Each resident wants the best possible schedule for himself/herself and many times not everybody can be accommodated. The chief resident may be held accountable.

However, there are some significant perks to the role. First and foremost, it can't hurt to have the words "chief resident" on your resume when you are applying for fellowships and later, attending radiology positions. Sometimes the chief may get to attend free conferences or may get an additional stipend at some programs. Other times, they benefit from getting inside information about the inner workings of the residency program before any other residents. And, occasionally it may help to get a position within the hospital or private practice where the residency is situated.

What Do We Look For In A Chief Resident?

The first and most important feature of a good chief resident is the ability to command respect among both the fellow residents and the attendings. We do not want to pick a resident that shows up late, gets involved in numerous conflicts with other attendings or residents, or who is not a "team player". Second, we look for a resident who has generally performed well academically and can handle the additional load of chief resident administrative responsibilities. And finally, we look for a chief resident who possesses a calm demeanor and is likable by all.

All these personality traits and features will allow the residency to continue to run smoothly and reduce the potential for significant conflict that can make the program director's job even more difficult. Also, it gives the program directors an additional "ear to the ground" and an advisor that can be extremely useful to prevent miscommunication.

What Makes The Decision To Find A Chief Resident Easy or Difficult?

Assessing who is to become chief is not a decision that is taken lightly. In fact, a very serious discussion ensues on a yearly basis among those that make the final decision. Some residency years, one or two academically high functioning residents have clearly been responsible for organizing the class and settling issues within the program. And, these same residents are also interested in performing the role and responsibilities of chief resident. When these stars align, the choice to make chief resident is very simple.

Other years, you have many interclass conflicts or there is no clear leader that makes decisions for the class. On occasion, we have a class with no one interested in performing the role of chief resident, knowing there are additional responsibilities. These factors can make it very difficult to come up with a final choice.

How Is The Chief Resident Finally Chosen?

Different programs have distinct policies regarding the installation of a new chief resident. At our program, the program directors choose the chief resident during the third year with input from fellow attendings and residents alike. The chief resident will typically begin his/her duties when the final year begins in July. Some years we have both educational and administrative chief radiology residents and other years we have had a single chief resident that takes care of both responsibilities. Other programs have a democratic policy with the residents forming a voting body that may vote for individual or multiple chief residents. The bottom line: there is no right or wrong way. But rather, the individual culture and traditions of the residency often determine how the choice of the chief resident is made.

"To Be or Not To Be" A Chief Resident

The chief resident has a significant role in the smooth running of a residency program. The responsibilities can be overwhelming for some and can be a great leadership opportunity for others. If you are chosen to be a chief resident, it is certainly an honor. But, it also involves a lot of extra work and hard choices. Make sure you are up to the task!!!

(1) https://www.aur.org/AnnualMeeting/

CHAPTER 21

Radiology Moonlighting: A Taboo?

● ● ●

RARELY DO CHAIRMEN AND RADIOLOGY program directors in academia utter the word "moonlighting" to their radiology residents, fellows, and employed attendings. Yet, moonlighting is a mainstay for many neophyte and seasoned radiologists. Why is the subject so taboo? Academic stakeholders want to know that their residents and practicing physicians are entirely dedicated to their primary responsibilities as learners and their duties at their daily jobs. To these stakeholders, moonlighting implies that their workers are employed in other endeavors that may "interfere" with their primary roles. Concerns such as duty hours and sleepiness during the day job can arise. Even worse, these workers can be perceived to be competing with the stakeholder's primary business.

But I would like to argue against both of these notions. First, it is unusual that the worker moonlights more than he/she can handle. Of course, anything taken to an extreme can be harmful to the practitioner. Too much sugar causes tooth decay. Too much water causes hyponatremia. And, too much moonlighting can theoretically be a distraction from the day job or training. However, it turns out that this impression of moonlighting is a widely perceived misconception.

I harken back to my days as a radiology resident and fellow. As a resident, I remember reading CT scans in a quiet room in the evening next to the CT technologist workstation, preliminarily providing initial interpretations by fax in order to satisfy the demands of the ER physician and provide coverage that otherwise would not ordinarily be available. I would also rapidly scan the plain films that were left over from the afternoon shift to make sure there were no impending disasters in the morning, occasionally detecting occult pneumothoraces, free air, pneumatosis, portal venous gas, and more. Instead of interfering with my role as a radiology resident at the time, I found the experience of moonlighting allowed me to read more quickly and accurately. It was supplemental to my day job and subsequently my career. In fact, my performance during my daytime residency position was enhanced by the extra practice of moonlighting. The ability to rapidly read films and scans quickly and accurately can only be achieved by the experience of having to do so. Moonlighting experience easily fits the bill.

Second, most moonlighting gigs are performed at a subsidiary of the primary institution or a local group that may need temporary coverage due to staffing needs. It would be certainly unusual for a moonlighter to "poach" cases from their primary residency program or his/her day job.

DISCORDANT VIEWS OF MOONLIGHTING- ACADEMICS VS. PRIVATE PRACTICE

Even more interesting, moonlighting is considered to be a badge of honor for the applicant to private practices to be displayed to the future employer of the moonlighter. In fact, when interviewing for private practice jobs, the stakeholders would specifically ask if I had done any moonlighting. For these private practice stakeholders, moonlighting implies that the trainee has the experience and wherewithal to handle the daily pressures of a bustling private radiology practice. This is a very different impression from the typical skeptical chairmen and residency directors.

Given the importance of moonlighting for a budding radiologist from both a training and future employment perspective, program directors should be actively discussing moonlighting instead of suppressing the information. Therefore, for the rest of this discussion, I am going to talk about where to find prime moonlighting experiences, what to avoid, and what you need to do prior to obtaining your first moonlighting gig.

WHERE DO I FIND MOONLIGHTING OPPORTUNITIES?

First of all, if you were fortunate enough to have a moonlighting opportunity embedded in your residency or fellowship program that is supported by the institution, then this is the best situation. You don't have to worry about "stepping on anyone's toes" and you will likely already be insured for the task. These opportunities are the simplest and best for the trainee.

I am aware, however, that many programs do not have these opportunities on hand. So, I would recommend you first ask either former or current residents and fellows about the opportunities in the local area. When you interview for your fellowship, make sure to get the phone number or email of the current fellows and ask them what they do for moonlighting. Usually, the current trainees know the local environment for moonlighting the best.

Let's say, however, the current residents or fellows are not moonlighting. What else could you do? You may want to call the local groups and find out if they have any temporary staffing needs. Many times the local group may need a warm body to "babysit" a magnet or give preliminary reads in the evening. This would be your opportunity...

Lastly, if all else fails, you may want either to search employment websites or to ask a locums company to help you find moonlighting opportunities. I would reserve this option for last because the companies that use these agencies are often charged a fee that may lower your pay rate.

WHAT MOONLIGHTING EXPERIENCES SHOULD I AVOID?

In the recent past, residents would finish their residency training, take and pass their oral boards, and then be board certified in radiology. No longer is this the case. This fact leads to some new technical issues with moonlighting as a fellow. In the past, I would have said by all means go ahead and give final reads as a moonlighting fellow. Instead nowadays as a typical radiology resident or fellow, I would consider reserving final reads until after you have passed your boards. Find moonlighting opportunities where you can give preliminary reads or be under the tutelage of a senior attending that is ultimately responsible for the final readings.

Why do I feel this way? Well, if you miss a finding and it goes to court, legally you may have a harder time defending your miss. If the plaintiff's attorney asks you if you were board certified at the time of the reading of the study and you say no, they can theoretically question your judgment at the time of the interpretation.

It is also important to check that your malpractice insurance for your residency or fellowship is compatible with the moonlighting site. If not, you should either obtain the correct insurance or the site should be off limits for the prospective candidate. If you are providing final reads for a practice or you don't have an occurrence policy, you should consider tail insurance.

Also, make sure that the time commitment to the moonlighting job is not too much. As discussed before, you certainly don't want your moonlighting to interfere with your day job.

What do I need to do prior to moonlighting?

1. Months prior to the prospect of moonlighting, you need to start getting the prep work done. The first thing to consider, make sure you get all the necessary state licenses that you may need. It can take a lot longer than you think to get a state medical license. Have all the paperwork ready.

2. Keep your CPR and ACLS certifications up to date. Some moonlighting opportunities require the applicant to have satisfied this requirement.

3. Prior to accepting any offer, make sure you feel comfortable with the requirements of the job. If they need someone to over read musculoskeletal MRI and you do not have experience with this, it is probably not the best situation for you. Be thorough when you ask the employer about what is required.

4. Let your residency or fellowship program know that you are going to be moonlighting. They need to be able to record your hours worked "off campus" as part of the duty hours requirement of the ACGME. If you are caught moonlighting without the knowledge of many programs, there could be a stiff penalty. It's probably not worth the risk of jeopardizing your residency or fellowship.

5. Once you have actually pinpointed the moonlighting opportunity, you then need to make sure your malpractice insurance will cover employment at the opportunity. Also, you must proceed rapidly with hospital credentialing, as this process can be very time-consuming. Hospital credentialing also includes sending off the malpractice insurance information to the hospital medical staff office.

Summary

Moonlighting can be a fantastic experience that supplements your residency and fellowship education. It can enhance your prospects for future employment, can allow you to gain speed and confidence at your daytime job, and let you more rapidly pay down your student debts. I highly recommend moonlighting if the opportunity is available, you are so inclined, and it is allowed by your residency or fellowship program.

Good references/links to find out more about moonlighting

(1) Moonlighting for Extra Money: Tempting, but Watch Out
http://www.medscape.com/viewarticle/761414

(2) Radiology resident moonlighting: A necessary evil?
http://www.auntminnie.com/index.aspx?sec=nws&sub=rad&pag=dis&ItemID=106972

Which Radiology Meeting Should I Attend?

● ● ●

A BIG DECISION NEEDS TO be made: At some programs, each resident can attend one academic conference during the 4 years of residency without having to present a poster or paper, all expenses paid. It may be toward the end of your tenure as a resident and time is running out to take advantage of the situation. You can "go big" and attend the largest radiology meeting out there- RSNA. (1) On the other hand, you may want to "go small" and consider a subspecialty meeting to delve into your area of interest. Or, perhaps you want to check out the academic meeting and hobnob with the faculty at the largest academic meeting- the AUR. (2) How do you make this difficult choice? Well, if you are in this enviable situation and need to make a decision, this article is for you!!!

"Going Big"- The RSNA

RSNA is the meeting that most radiology residents decide to attend. It is a meeting that has "something for everyone", literally. Traditionally, the RSNA is by far the largest of all radiology meetings and covers every subspecialty within radiology. But this also presents a problem: how do you decide on what to attend when you are there? Because of the vast size of the conference, I would recommend that if you decide to go, you need a roadmap prior to arriving at the conference. Know what meetings, poster presentations, or other areas of interest you are going to attend prior to arriving. If you do not outline a plan prior to arriving, you will likely miss half of the more relevant, informative, and interesting presentations since the conference is so enormous and the different activities can be far, far away from one another.

In addition, if you are in the process of studying for the core examination and the timing is right to attend a conference, this may be the conference for you. There are usually loads of activities for residents including review courses that may be helpful for the resident scheduled to take his/her boards. Possibly even more important than the review course itself, you will also be able to network with other residents in a similar situation, giving you an opportunity to learn the best resources to study for examinations as well as learn about other programs throughout the country. In many practices, at least one attending from your group will be present at this conference. This also allows the resident to take advantage of dinners or other engagements scheduled with vendors.

The one big disadvantage of a conference like this one: it tends to be a bit more impersonal than some of the smaller conferences that are available. For the radiology resident, this may not be an issue, depending on your fellow attendees and how you schedule your days.

"going small"- The Subspecialty Conference

My preference is for this sort of conference. I usually attend the <u>Society of Nuclear Medicine Conference</u> (3) every other year, an example of a particular subspecialty conference. I find that these conferences are the best for learning the intimate details of a particular subspecialty. The newest information in subspecialties tends to get presented for the first time in these subspecialty conferences.

If you are interested in a particular subspecialty and want to choose a fellowship in the area of the conference, going to these subspecialty meetings is often times the best method of networking to get to know the physicians in the subspecialty. These conferences offer this possibility because they are smaller and give more of a "feeling of camaraderie" since the members of the conference tend to be more engaged in specific subspecialty activities.

AUR Meeting- The Academic Radiology Conference

Every year in our program, our chief resident is allowed to participate in this conference. It is a wonderful conference to find out the state of academic radiology throughout the country from a resident perspective as they have specific programs available for the chief residents. As a program director, I also tend to go to this conference once per year in order to keep up with the changes in radiology academics on a yearly basis.

In addition to the potential relevance, the conference is not so large that you can get lost in a meeting like the RSNA. In fact, you can easily get to know the players in the academic world. I would highly recommend this conference if you are interested in academics or are the chief resident in your residency program. Residents attending this conference obtain an invaluable source of information about all residency programs throughout the United States that they can share with their resident colleagues when they return.

The "Pure" Board Review/CME Conference

Lastly, there is the board review or CME conference. Usually, these conferences are dedicated to either board review or a specific topic/selection of topics. In our residency program, many residents attend local board review courses prior to taking the core exam. It is a good resource as a means to review the information learned from studying.

Other sorts of CME conferences are also widely available throughout the United States and abroad. Typically, the attendees of these conferences are more likely to be fully trained radiologists who want to learn more about a particular subspecialty or area of interest and/or may want to travel to a particular destination. (I recently went to a conference at Disney World like this to learn about digital breast tomography!) That being said, the topics covered by these conferences are usually already present in some form or another in a radiology residency program, so the yield of this conference for the radiology resident may be slightly lower. From my experience, most trainees that attend these conferences are stationed at the institution responsible for the conference.

Summary Statement About Conferences During Residency

Like almost everything else in this world, one size does not fit all when deciding to attend a conference. RSNA is a good introduction to the world of conferences as it is the largest and the most general. Subspecialty conferences are great for networking, especially if you are interested in a fellowship or a particular subspecialty. The AUR meeting is an excellent option for academic sorts and chief residents. And finally, board reviews/CME conferences are a great tool to review studies for the boards/core examination. Lots of decisions to make and so little time... Hopefully, this article will give another perspective on how to make this big decision!

(1) http://www.rsna.org/Annual_Meeting.aspx

(2) https://www.aur.org/AnnualMeeting/

(3) http://www.snmmi.org/AM/index.aspx?ItemNumber=12337

CHAPTER 23

Best Radiology Electives For The Senior Resident

● ● ●

It's GETTING TOWARD THE END of your 3rd year and you are studying intensely for your core examination. All of a sudden, you get a phone call from your chief resident. He says, " We are making the schedule for next year. What would you like to do for your senior year electives?" You realize you haven't really thought this through and you are not sure what to do. He just assigns you to a standard fourth-year schedule.

Believe it or not, this is a situation that often happens to most residents. Choosing your fourth-year electives is not a decision you should take lightly. You should not have the choice made for you, nor should you make a choice without really thinking deeply about what you want. Your senior year elective choices can have repercussions upon your comfort zones in private practice and also your practice patterns for years to come. So, today we are going to discuss what not to do when you decide upon your senior schedule, which standard rotations are the best for senior electives and some innovative ideas for creating rotations on your fourth-year schedule that will really enhance your residency education and your career.

WHICH FOURTH YEAR ELECTIVES SHOULD YOU AVOID?

When you create a schedule for your fourth year, I would highly recommend avoiding adding scheduled rotations that duplicate your fellowship. Several times as associate residency director, I have had requests from residents to do a half a year in mammography when the resident has already been selected for a mammography fellowship. What's the point in that? In our residency program and many residency programs throughout the country, it is important to remember that 90 percent of residents eventually do private practice and only 10 percent work in academia. So, chances are you will not be working only within your specialty. In fact, according to **many articles** (1,2,3), most radiology job descriptions want the new radiologist to not only practice in one subspecialty but also to cover other areas of radiology. So, if you decide to do a half-year in the subspecialty of your fellowship, you are decreasing the opportunity to learn subspecialties outside of your comfort zone. And, you are also decreasing your desirability for being hired by a private practice.

For instance, if there are two candidates, one that wants to do only mammography, and another that feels comfortable reading MSK MRI as well as being sub-specialized in mammography, which candidate is going to be chosen by a private practice? It's rather simple. It's almost always the one that can do both. You are missing out on a potential opportunity if you choose to duplicate your fellowship.

Also, I would avoid choosing too many mini-fellowships that are within your comfort zone. If you feel like you are a great musculoskeletal MRI reader, it doesn't make sense to do too many additional rotations in the same subspecialty. In private practice, you generally do not want to pigeon hole yourself into only a few subspecialty areas. A series of fourth-year electives or "mini-fellowships" in areas that you are well versed will limit the time you have to learn other subspecialties outside of your areas of comfort. Time not spent on remediating areas of weakness during your last year of residency will ultimately prevent you from practicing comfortably in these "weaker" subspecialty areas when you are an attending radiologist.

THE CONVENTIONAL FOURTH YEAR ELECTIVE APPROACH

If you are going down the conventional route of fourth year electives, there are two routes I would choose. First, it would be reasonable to select an emphasis in an area that you are interested but in which you are not doing your fellowship. Since you will be completing these electives fairly close in time to your search for full-time radiologist work, this will allow you to have a second area of subspecialty confidence and diversify your competencies when you are looking for work.

Second, I would choose electives in areas of weakness. Residency is the time to get to know the different subspecialties and get your hands dirty. The more competent you are in all aspects of radiology, the more desirable you will be for private practices. It behooves the budding radiologist to get to the point of basic competency in as many areas as possible.

The Unconventional Fourth Year Elective Choice

What is the difference between a good and a great radiologist? It's pretty simple. A good radiologist can generally make the correct imaging calls. A great radiologist can make the correct call, understands the deep clinical significance of the call, and can predict the subsequent patient outcomes. If I had to redo my residency over again, I would choose the unconventional radiology elective approach to correlate the imaging with the practical to further deepen these great clinical radiology qualities.

So, how do you arrange an elective choice such as this? It definitely will take a bit more work on the part of the radiology resident and you will have to go out of your way to communicate with other specialty directors, but it really pays to arrange a few weeks or a month rotating on a medical or surgical rotation with correlative imaging. For example, if you were interested in musculoskeletal radiology, I would highly recommend calling the surgical director of orthopedics and ask him/her if you can watch and participate in the clinical workup of patients, orthopedic surgeries, and the subsequent follow-up of patients. Then, when you work up a patient that has had a medial meniscal tear, you will have seen the surgery and the aftercare follow-up of these patients. You will really understand how the imaging fits into the equation and the significance of your imaging calls. I guarantee the learning that you get from an elective such as this will stick with you for the rest of your radiology career.

I would also recommend to wash, rinse, and repeat. If you can arrange this sort of elective in multiple subspecialties, whether in orthopedics, neurosurgery/neurology, breast surgery, oncology, cardiothoracic surgery, pulmonology, vascular surgery, obstetrics/gynecology, or whatever other clinical subspecialties interest you, it would be a highly effective way to have a great diverse overall fourth year experience that will last a lifetime. In addition, you will have a clinical knowledge of the imaged patient that most other radiologists do not have.

Final Thoughts About Fourth Year Electives

The fourth year of radiology residency is a time to explore in more depth the subspecialties that you have encountered during your first three years. Because you are so close to becoming a board certified practicing radiologist, the fourth year elective takes on a particularly important significance since the subjects that are learned will make a difference in your clinical practice. So, please pay attention to creating a great fourth-year elective experience. Don't squander the opportunity!!!

(1) http://www.diagnosticimaging.com/practice-management/double-fellowship-new-standard-radiology

(2) http://www.jacr.org/article/S1546-1440(15)00522-0/abstract

(3) http://www.jacr.org/article/S1546-1440(15)00956-4/abstract

CHAPTER 24

The Difficult Radiology Attending

● ● ●

IF YOU EVER APPLY FOR a residency, fellowship, or a full-fledged radiology position, and the interviewers claim all the staff is perfect, run away, and run away fast! (Of course, our program is perfect!!) Just like any other profession, school, or body of people, not all people are pleasant. Anyone that tells you otherwise is sincerely lying. Fortunately, most individuals in the radiology profession have stable friendly personalities. But, in any room of 100 people, you will have psychopaths(1 out of 100) (1), narcissists, border-line personalities (6 out of 100) (2), and many other personality types. And, radiology is likely no different. During your radiology residency, these issues are magnified because you have to sit for a concentrated amount of time with this person. In fact, it could be for hours at a time. So, you need to learn coping mechanisms to deal with these people. Ironically, I found that some of these most difficult attending personalities lent themselves to my best and most intense learning experiences. It's where I learned to develop a thick skin, become more of an independent radiologist, tightened my dictation style, and learned to listen. These were the formative years for me. If you think of the tough individual as another link in the chain of learning experiences, most of these days, weeks, or months that you sit with this difficult attending will seem to have more relevance to your overall education. Your time spent will certainly not be perfect but will be much improved. This segment is going to go through 12 different personality types that you may encounter during your residency program and teach you how you can use each personality type to add to your body of experience and build you into a successful and excellent radiologist.

The Narcissist

Everyone knows this individual. I personally always think of that main character from <u>Dragon's Lair</u> (Dirk the Daring) (3), always with the perfect hair, the expensive clothes, and showing off his skills (or lack thereof!!!) to the world. As they say, "God's Gift to Humanity". These individuals will often appear overconfident and some will make fools of themselves. It's going to be the attending that never uses liver windows because he says he can always easily detect all liver lesions in soft tissue windows. He's just too good to make that extra effort. What's great about working with these sorts during your residency training? When you are done with a rotation with this individual, you will learn how to avoid being overconfident and look more carefully in places that the narcissist will miss due to overconfidence. Most important, it is a great time to learn how to be humble, an important feature of a good radiologist. The best quote to describe this sort of individual is "Often wrong but never in doubt." Radiologists cannot <u>always</u> be right!!!

The Know It All

If you were in school, this would be the talkative kid that is always raising his hand. Or think of Hermione from the <u>Harry Potter Series</u> (4)... This person can be extremely annoying but smart and well versed. The know-it-all gives the resident a distinct learning experience but usually takes the thunder away from something that another attending or you may have discovered. As a resident, you have a lot to learn from this person. He or she will teach you all sorts of things in radiology that others will not and give you a sense of humility.

The Absent Attending

You know this type of individual, always leaving the department at the drop of the hat. He/she expects you to do all the work for them during the day. And, the person is rarely available when you have important questions. I have found that this experience is probably one of the best learning experiences you can have as a resident. It allows you to take charge of a rotation that you normally would be merely following. You will need to look up lots of information on Google and ask other residents/attendings what to do. In fact, when you are done with the rotation with this sort of attending, you will be able to run the department because you will be able to handle most of the day-to-day issues on your own, related to your experience of having the unavailable attending!

THE SMITTEN ATTENDING (WITH SOMEONE ELSE!)

So, you are working in your interventional rotation and your co-resident or medical student is very handsome or pretty. Your attending does not seem to want to listen to anything you have to say. The "boss" always goes to the other resident to teach them, asks them questions, and forgets about you. What do you do? Well, the answer is simple. You work twice as hard to get their attention. Working hard on this rotation, may not pay off in terms of getting a recommendation from this individual, but it will allow you to put your heart and soul into your work and make the rotation an intense work experience, one that may be more similar to breathing and living the subspecialty rotation. When you go into practice, you will be thankful for the extra time and experience that you may not have had otherwise!!!

THE OBSESSIVELY DETAIL ORIENTED ATTENDING

When you come back from dictating a case, this is the sort of attending that will mince every word and tell you why each word and phrase should have been different. Don't take offense at this sort of mentor. Most of the time they mean well. But, the experience of having to write the same dictation over and over; overcorrecting every statement until you make it the way he/she wants can be painful. But, dictation is one of the more difficult elements in radiology to master. So, this experience can be invaluable for honing your reports and making them much stronger and exacting. Believe it or not, consider this person a resource to make your future reports that much better!

The Sociopath

Watch your back! He/she will typically seem to be the nicest attending in the whole department. In fact, the radiologist often times will tell you exactly what you want to hear. Until, Wham! You find out at the end of the month that your evaluation from the program director is not what it originally seemed. The sociopath will not tell you about what he/she thought of you at the time of your rotation and takes pride in stealthily making the life of the radiology resident miserable. The good news is the rotation will seem to be just fine when you are there. It is only the afterglow that causes the misery. But your experience with this sort of attending will teach you an invaluable experience; never assume that everything is ok. Always, ask and find out what you can improve and how you can do things better. This experience is a wake-up call for the naive resident!

Dr. Bizarre

Out of all the radiology personality types, believe it or not, you will find this one to be one of the most interesting. I can remember one of my former attendings telling me about a mentor who was constantly drooling when he spoke and whose eyes were incessantly tearing. He stood at the mere height of 4 foot 3. But, when you actually spoke to this person, the passion for teaching and his profession shone through everything. These attendings tend to have some of the most diverse backgrounds and interests. When you actually treat these folks as mentors/teachers, you find that they have very memorable ideas and behaviors that you would not learn from the more typical personality/appearance. I have incorporated many of their teachings into my daily practice and have found that their teachings tend to stick because of the unusual delivery and presentation. Typically, you will remember fondly the days that you work with these people and have good stories to tell as well!

The Dictator

You will find this attending demanding and tough. He treats all his staff with an iron fist. This radiologist will appear unreasonable at times and expects everyone- nurses, technologist, and residents- to bow toward every whim. Unfortunately, you will need to do the same or expect his wrath. The environment may at times be unpleasant and you will need a thick skin, but I have found that these attendings make the residents more rigorous in their approach to running a department, adopting search patterns, and learning radiology. Use this opportunity to incorporate the dictator's demands into your routine, and I can assure you will become a much better radiologist!

The Gossiper/Talker

You will have some of the best conversations with this attending and will learn about every character in the department. This person talks a lot and can prevent staff from getting their work done. And, some of the information you may or may not have wanted to know. However, listen to this person very carefully because they can be a great source of information about what is really going on in the department, a very valuable commodity. My advice to you is to reveal only what you want revealed to this attending or else your story may become publicized as well!

The Inappropriate Attending

Most people know this type of personality. He/she may yell at the patients, make off-color jokes with the wrong sorts of people, or may get a little too touchy/feely. To this day, I use these uncomfortable situations to be instructive of what not to do as an attending radiologist. In fact, I use these experiences as ways to remember to model good behaviors to my residents by the allegories/stories that have occurred!!!

The Loner

Many residents feel the need to get instantaneous feedback from their attendings. This attending will not only give you any feedback; he/she may not even talk to you during your shared time. You may be "pulling teeth" to get this attending to teach and talk to you. You may feel like you are always being observed and assessed, but with no response. Remember that the world of radiology is not always a specialty of instantaneous feedback. You may find out what you have done right or wrong months or maybe years afterward. This attending personality type truly prepares you for the real world!

THE UNINTELLIGIBLE RADIOLOGIST

Most residents know this type. It's the attending with tons of typos in their reports and with clinicians that are constantly calling this attending to figure out what he reported in his radiology impressions. So what is the big advantage to having an attending like this? Well, you are going to need to learn how to field the clinician's questions about his cases in a thoughtful intelligent manner without incriminating its author. It's a great way to solidify your radiology impressions and learn to communicate with the clinicians!!!

THE BOTTOM LINE

There are all sorts of personalities that radiology residents will encounter during their 4 years of training. I have probably just scratched the surface. Tough personalities can lead to trying times on a daily, weekly, or monthly basis. However, the experiences that you will have can be invaluable in your development as a radiology resident. Use these personalities to enhance your reputation and skills as a radiologist. Don't let these difficult attendings get the best of you!!!

(1) http://www.livescience.com/7859-psychopath-answers-remain-elusive. html

(2) https://www.bpdcentral.com/faq/personality-disorders

(3) https://en.wikipedia.org/wiki/Dragon%27s_Lair

(4) https://en.wikipedia.org/wiki/Harry_Potter_and_the_Philosopher% 27s_Stone

The Struggling Radiology Resident

● ● ●

IN ANY PROFESSION OR CAREER, some employees lag the performance of their peers. It turns out that radiology residency is no different from any other job in this respect. The key, however, is for either the employer to be able to identify the struggling worker or for the employee to recognize that he or she is struggling. It is only when this process happens that interventions can occur. In addition, it is important for this process of identification to be early and effective. The goal of the radiology program is to help these residents along as soon as possible to allow early and more effective remediation. Early remediation can prevent the further downward spiral of a struggling resident that could lead to probation, suspension, or even worse, job loss. On occasion, there is no effective remediation for certain individuals, but that is the exception rather than the rule. No matter how you slice it, loss of a resident is devastating for both the radiology program and the radiology resident alike. So, my goal for this chapter's discussion is geared toward the individual struggling radiology resident in order to prevent him/her from going down this pathway. We will discuss how to identify oneself as struggling, what you can do to intervene prior to more serious repercussions, and how to deal with your attendings and colleagues when you are the "struggling resident".

SELF-IDENTIFICATION

As is said, a problem cannot be fixed unless you know a problem exists. So, self-identification of oneself as struggling becomes crucial. Some residents know from the very beginning that they are having difficulties and have good insight into their situation. Others may be having difficulties but are not aware. In addition, sometimes the feedback that residents get from attendings, technologists, nurses, and administrators can be different from the truth and outright misleading. Given that radiology residents tend to have limited responsibilities during their first year of residency, this issue is more likely to go unnoticed during this first formative year of residency. So, we will first talk briefly about what may be some of the indicators that you are struggling during your residency.

I am also going to classify the reasons for the struggling resident as either academic or professional in order to simplify and organize the discussion. Let's first start by talking about some of the indicators that a resident may be struggling in academics.

How to Know If You Are Struggling Academically

Noon conference can be an excellent time to discover your position relative to your colleagues. If you notice that you are unable to answer questions that are easily answered by your colleagues on a consistent basis: it can be a red flag. If you have a hard time describing or making a finding on studies geared to the first year resident most of the time, you may be struggling. If different attendings giving noon conference consistently become frustrated with your answers, you may want to consider that you are struggling.

Readouts with your attending may help to self-determine whether you are struggling. Are you able to answer routine questions appropriately? Is an attending that typically accepts resident dictations re-dictating everything you write? Is there a sense of frustration from your supervisor? Do your attendings provide you with some sense of independence during procedures similar to others in your program? These are some hints that all may not be quite right.

Next, think about your experiences on "buddy call". Do you feel comfortable going over films with your colleagues, attendings, and other clinicians? Is there a sense of frustration from these people with your reads?

Are attendings not really satisfied when they find out they are on call with you?

How about feedback and evaluations? Is the feedback you receive from attendings routinely negative? Are milestone evaluations always below par? Do you receive comments from attendings that are always negative?

You might think that the in-service exam would also be a good metric of resident performance. But, it turns out as associate program director; I put much less faith in academic evaluations based upon the in-service examination. I have found a poor correlation with resident academic performance. So as a resident, I would not rely upon this form of self-assessment. However, in combination with the in-service exam, if you are underperforming on other residency based quizzes or examinations, this can be an indicator of true academic issues.

How to Know If You Are Struggling Professionally

This area can be harder to recognize for the struggling resident. Many don't realize they have a problem until it's too late. But, we will go through some examples that you may be able to self-identify.

Absentia in its many forms is a leading indicator of professionalism based struggles. Are you routinely late to conferences and readouts and do you sense the frustration in others? Do your colleagues too often have to cover for you because you are not available? Have you been cited multiple times for missing conferences or required meetings?

Conflicts with classmates and colleagues can be a prominent indicator of professionalism struggles. Are there routine yelling matches with your fellow residents? Do your colleagues not want to help you out with call coverage, studying, or other routine residency issues? Are you routinely fighting with the secretaries, nurses, technologists, or even attendings?

Substance abuse is all too common a cause for having a difficult residency. Take a serious look at your habits and if they may be truly affecting your performance. Are you routinely using alcohol or other illicit substances?

Chronic disease can be a cause for day-to-day residency struggles. Cancer, hepatitis, infectious diseases are all problems that can cause fatigue and difficulty with concentrating on a long shift.

And of course, there are psychological issues such as depression, anxiety, schizophrenia, and more. These issues are more likely to go unnoticed by the afflicted resident. But some residents, already diagnosed with these disorders, may have better insight. These residents need to take a hard look and see if these problems are affecting their residency performance.

SELF-INTERVENTIONS

So, the next step in the process is to figure out how to remedy the situation prior to bigger repercussions. If you know your issues are academic or professional, you can certainly take measures to stem the riptide. We will go through several of these avenues.

You've decided that you're struggling academically. What do you do? The next step is to make a realistic assessment of why you are struggling. For some people, it may be the quantity and for others, it may be the quality of their studies.

1. QUANTITY OF LEARNING

Having been through the residency process and supervised many residents over the years, I have learned that radiology is a reading intensive specialty and in order to increase one's knowledge base, a resident needs to create a means to be able to cover all the important and relevant topics within the residency program. So, the first question is: what do you base your study schedule on? Some residents will use the curriculum guidelines from their residency program. Others will split the ABR core exam (1) topics into bits of information that they can review. Even others may use STATDx/Radprimer (2) to guide their studying. The bottom line is that you need to find some guideline that will allow you to cover all the topics that you need to know.

The second question: have you created a schedule for yourself that will allow you to cover the necessary topics during residency and what are some options for the resident? Many residents don't realize the amount they need to learn in order to become a proficient radiologist. A schedule therefore becomes very important for the struggling resident. The schedule can vary from one person to the next. Some people do better with studying for short blocks of time. Others prefer to slog it out for a long block at once. It doesn't matter how you complete the necessary work, whether you take 2, 3, or 4, topics per evening, but the work needs to get completed. A regimented schedule will allow you to go through the appropriate information for each rotation.

2. Quality of Learning

The next step is to assess if it is how you are studying that is the problem. Some residents study for hours every night, only to find that their knowledge base is not up to par. You would think that by the time one gets into the radiology specialty, they would have a method for studying well. But, that is certainly not the case for many residents. Studying and reading for the radiology resident is very different from studying for medical school classes and the boards. Radiology emphasizes pictures. Medical schools emphasize words.

So, if you are truly studying for hours at nighttime without result, try studying differently. I would recommend emphasizing reading the pictures and captions within a book instead of the general text. Many residents do not realize they need to do this in order to be a more effective radiology student.

You may also want to explore case review series over general text reading. Again, pictures are the center of the radiologist's world. I find that a general text helps more when you have experienced a case firsthand during the daytime and you want to find out more. On the other hand, a case image with text is more similar to the day-to-day work of the radiologist and will allow many residents to digest the information better.

There is one last item that I want to bring to light. On occasion, a radiology residency may make a learning disability evident. Because radiology is different than other subspecialties and the methods for studying differ from other areas as well, some residents have problems with the transition. Some residents have problems looking at a picture and translating the picture into findings and conclusions. It is not something that is usually tested prior to beginning radiology. If you think that this may be your situation, it behooves these residents to consider psychological testing to better find a more effective means of studying. Dollars spent to solve this issue now if you do have a learning disability, may pay itself back in spades later on.

Fixing Professionalism

Professional issues and their solutions can vary widely. For the absentee resident, it may be as simple as creating and sticking to a schedule to make sure he/she attends all the necessary events on time. If you are in constant conflict with your colleagues, you may need to learn to relate to others better. This may involve sharing more or not be taking everything to heart. On the other hand, maybe the conflicts are related to other more serious issues such as substance abuse or health problems. The important thing to remember: there are many sources of help for the radiology resident. Whether it is your colleagues, attendings, program directors, chairman, the Physician Assistance Program, a psychiatrist, or other interventions, there is someone at your program that can support you. It is very important to talk to someone if there is a professionalism issue that needs to be addressed. And, there is always help if the situation becomes unbearable.

How to Deal With Attendings and Colleagues If You Are Struggling

OK. So you have identified that you are struggling and you have created the means to effectively remedy the issues. The next problem is that you may have created an environment where the expectations of your colleagues are so low that it may be very difficult to defy their expectations. I like to describe this as the "vicious circle". Everything that you do is now going to be much more scrutinized than your colleagues. Even though your performance may improve to the level of your colleagues, it may not be recognized and may still be perceived as below par. This is probably the most difficult part of being an underperforming resident. So, what do you do at this point?

I would recommend continuing with the remediation program at hand. Healing a reputation takes not a few days or months. Rather, it can take years. Eventually, your effort will be recognized, but it is not without a lot of work and effort. You will have to suffer through some of the expectations of your attendings and colleagues until they realize you are a capable resident. This process takes grit and determination. You are going to have to ignore the expectations of others and create your own expectations for yourself. Eventually, you will notice a change in how you are treated, but remember, it will not happen overnight.

Summary

Radiology residency is a big transition for most residents, and some may really struggle at the beginning academically or professionally. If you are struggling at this time in your life, don't let these shortcomings define you. The measure of greatness is how you overcome obstacles such as completing a radiology residency, a major achievement. Struggling radiology residents often become radiology attendings with greater empathy for the struggles of others and can become the most successful radiologists.

(1) https://www.theabr.org/sites/all/themes/abr-media/pdf/CORE_Exam_Study_Guide_FINAL%28V11%29.pdf

(2) http://www.radprimer.com

CHAPTER 26

The Other Struggling Radiology Residents

● ● ●

A RADIOLOGY RESIDENCY PROGRAM IS like a family. When one person is afflicted academically or professionally, all of its members suffer down the road. Just as important as it is to be aware of and help the struggling radiology resident, it is also important to remember that one struggling resident can have serious repercussions on the remainder of the radiology residency program. It is not just the program director and chairman that reap the consequences of the struggling resident. Often times unfairly, it is the class members that take up much of the additional burden, whether it be extra call shifts, less time spent on educational rotations, uncomfortable personality conflicts, or extra time spent educating the failing resident. So, this post is dedicated to the other radiology residents that are affected by the struggling radiology resident. First, we will go through how other residents can appropriately identify and help the struggling resident and possibly get this person to the attention of the program director. Then we will go through what a resident should and should not do when there is a resident struggling either academically or professionally. And finally, we will examine how the residency program should commit its resources toward the struggling resident vs. the other radiology residents.

IDENTIFICATION OF STRUGGLING RESIDENT BY COLLEAGUES

Many times the first residency program members to notice that a resident is struggling is not the program director, chairman, or attendings, but rather the struggling resident's fellow colleagues. Fellow residents are more likely to interact with the struggling resident on a social basis in a more comfortable setting where the struggling resident is more likely to discuss his/her issues. This is an opportunity to learn more about how your fellow classmate is feeling about residency. He/she may even ask for your help. My advice is: give whatever help is reasonable to your classmate so that they can perform well. Residency is not a competition, but rather a team environment. In addition, the help that you give your fellow struggling resident will come back to you many times over. Whether you decide to teach your colleague or help them out with other residency issues, you will find that you will learn more about your material and yourself. Even better, you may be able to stem a progressive downward spiral to probation or even worse, a point where you and your classmates would suffer more dire consequences.

Sometimes the identification of the struggling resident may be a bit more subtle than a simple comment to you about their struggles. Different from an attending that sees a resident on a noon conference or on a single day, you as a fellow resident may notice a pattern of taking cases and missing all the findings each time or multiple absences that are not recorded by the program. Or you may notice bad habits such as drinking a little too much, something a little bit off, or a strange affect. These can be important sentinel events and you may want to address the issue with your program director or chairman to make sure the struggling resident gets the help that he/she needs.

In the end, it really pays to identify the struggling resident. Remember... It often affects not just that resident, but the entire program as well.

How Can The Residents Help With The Academically Struggling Resident?

It is the primary responsibility of the program directors, attendings, and chairman to handle the academically struggling radiology resident. But, for the struggling resident's rehabilitation to succeed, the program often needs to have the participation of all. In fact, the role of the other residents can be the key to the stability of the program through this trying time as well as be increasing the likelihood that the struggling resident will eventually succeed.

Prior to any remediation, it is important to determine if the struggling resident is willing to accept the help of the other members of the program. So, the role of the other residents can only begin when the struggling resident asks for help from his/her fellow colleagues. You certainly cannot force a struggling resident to participate in remediation efforts if the struggling resident is not willing or able.

If you remember the previous chapter- The Struggling Radiology Resident, we discussed how the academically struggling radiology resident might have difficulty with coping with the quantity or quality of his/her work. So, I will go over briefly how the other residents should attend to each of these issues.

For a struggling resident that is unable to schedule an appropriate time for studying, what should his/her colleagues do? This becomes a time management issue. It would be appropriate to help the struggling resident to create his/her own schedule. Sometimes it helps just to sit down with the struggling resident and show them how you schedule your study time and what you have been reading on each rotation.

In the case of a struggling resident that has difficulty with the quality of studying, it would make sense to have group study time and to present cases to one another in order to improve taking cases. Or, it may be a good idea to go over questions with all the residents to practice testing skills. These processes not only help the struggling resident but may be good practice for the entire team.

How Can Fellow Residents Help With The Professionally Struggling Radiology Resident?

When it comes to a professionally struggling resident, the fellow residents have to be a bit more careful with assisting in interventions. Obviously, the intervention will depend on the primary cause of professionalism problems.

For the resident that is often absent, it may be possible to address this issue by simply asking the resident where they have been or why they have not been around in a non-confrontational manner. Sometimes the struggling resident may not be aware of the burden he/she is placing on the other residents. This may make this resident aware of the issues he is causing and take responsibility for his actions. Again, if this does not work, it may just be as important to bring the issue to the program's attention.

For the resident with personality issues, whether it is a resident that is abusive or a resident that is unengaged, you need to be a bit more careful. If you are friendly with this resident, by all means, it does not hurt to find out if there is an overall cause for the behavior. But be careful to not be overly intrusive as it may not be appropriate to get involved much further. Certainly, if the struggling resident is amenable to helpful suggestions of conflict resolution within the residency, talk to this person about some of these issues in an appropriate setting. Or, it may be appropriate to make a suggestion to this resident to seek professional help if the resident is amenable.

In many programs at one time or another, just like the general population, some struggling residents will experience psychiatric issues or may be involved with alcohol or illicit drug use. These situations can be extremely touchy. Many of these residents may not have insight into their problems and are more likely to refuse help from colleagues or attendings. Of course, a few may have insight. But, if you notice a struggling resident with one of these issues, it is usually best to bring the issue to the attention of the program director or chairman of the department so that they can get the resident into the appropriate channels for treatment. However, there are exceptions to every rule. And on occasion, the struggling resident's colleagues may have intimate knowledge of the resident and may be more likely to be able to get the resident appropriate help. But, be careful in this situation because there are occasional unforeseen legal and professional ramifications for the caring colleague. A resident without insight into his/her problems may see this helpful resident as antagonistic and can theoretically pursue these channels.

How to Commit the Program's Resources Toward The Struggling Resident

Over my tenure as associate residency director, I have learned that dealing with the issues of a struggling resident can be a drain on a program's administration and resources. The time that is normally spent toward improving the residency program instead needs to be placed on the issues of the one resident. Especially in smaller programs with less faculty and monetary resources, the time spent can overwhelm the program directors, chairman, and heads of Graduate Medical Education. While it is important that the struggling resident gets the necessary help and remediation, we have to remember that other residents also need to have a functional residency program. It is easy to forget about the other residents in this process. So, it is the residency director and chairman's role to place additional efforts to concentrate on not just the struggling resident, but the other residents at these times and to make sure the residency program continues to run smoothly.

Back To The Other Residents

Every program at one time or another will have a struggling resident. And, it is important for fellow resident colleagues to help out if possible with the identification and remediation of the struggling resident. But, it is often the other residents that suffer most from the consequences of a struggling resident's actions and inactions as well as the choices that the administration makes to help the struggling resident. So, everyone involved needs to make a concerted effort to not forget about the struggling resident's colleagues. Or else, these residents can truly become the "other struggling residents".

CHAPTER 27

The Uncooperative Patient- The Radiology Resident's View

● ● ●

As a <u>RADIOLOGY RESIDENT</u>, THE patient experience differs greatly from other specialty services. Typically, he or she sees a patient for a solitary encounter or even less commonly, a second or third chance episode. Rarely does the radiology resident have continual exposure to the same patient. He/she has limited time to interact with the patients, even more so than other clinicians. Therefore, the radiology resident does not often establish deep connections with patients like other specialties. So, we have to view our experience through a very different lens.

In our "radiology world", all of us will be involved in one of these dilemmas: The patient may refuse to drink barium, deny the imaging department the crucial second portion of a test, physically combat the staff, refuse procedure consent, move during a study, or be noncompliant with our instructions. In these situations, we often do not have the full picture of why the patient may not be cooperating. So in this discussion, I will go through how you, as radiology residents, establish a rapport with these patients to motivate the patient to complete a test. Also, I will discuss a couple of typical situations with "uncooperative" patients that you may encounter and how you can prevent them from escalating from bad to worse.

PATIENT RAPPORT AND MOTIVATION

As a human being, I can think of nothing less motivating than doing something for someone that I don't know and for a reason that I don't understand. Many times, this is exactly the situation that the patient is experiencing. The patient is often brought down to our department without a clue as to what test they are having with people they don't know. They may be placed in confined quarters with minimal if any human interaction.

Think about it... Imagine coming down from one of the floors to have a procedure such as a barium enema and seeing someone without any identification whatsoever. As a patient, I can picture the thoughts going through his/her head. Is this person qualified to do the procedure? Am I going to be butchered by someone I don't even know? Patients in this situation can often feel dehumanized and vulnerable. How can we minimize this poor patient experience? The first step is very simple: introduce yourself. Who are you and why are you there? This alone can motivate a patient to complete a study.

Secondly, explain the procedure. I have found that taking the time out to simply explain a procedure will often times go a long way to diffusing a potentially intense situation. Not only does explaining the procedure make the patient more comfortable and knowledgeable about his/her own care, but it also establishes that you are a professional that will be competent to perform a procedure.

And finally, let the patient know if you are going to be the one that is performing the procedure and, if not, at least you will be around to monitor him/her when the procedure is occurring. What a relief to know that there is someone in the department that has his/her back!

A COUPLE OF SPECIAL SITUATIONS
THE COMBATIVE PATIENT/FAMILY

So, you are on interventional radiology for the month and are on your fourth consent for the evening prior to finishing up with your work. In the back of your mind, you are thinking that you are soon finally going home. You enter the room and introduce yourself to the patient and daughter. Subsequently, you start to discuss a PICC line consent that you have planned for tomorrow's morning procedures and you begin to rattle off the risks, alternatives, and benefits to the procedure. As the discussion ensues, you notice on the door of the room a sign saying feeding precautions: Severe Risk of Aspiration- Do Not Feed the Patient! You then look back to the patient/daughter and notice that the daughter is rapidly shoveling food from home into the patient's mouth. You halt the discussion and say to the daughter, "You really shouldn't be feeding your Mom. She has aspiration precautions and can choke on the food that you are giving her..." The daughter yells back, "How Dare YOU Tell Me How to Treat My Mom. She Has Not Eaten For Days And I Will Give Her What She Wants!!!!" The patient then begins to cry and the daughter gets right up into your face in a threatening way as if she is going to punch you in the face.

How would you deal with a real world possible situation such as this? There are several options. But, as the radiology resident with limited knowledge of the patient's situation, you need to treat it a bit differently than a primary care doctor or a specialist that sees the patient every day.

As the radiology resident, of course, you first need to make sure to de-escalate the situation. You do not continue to argue with the patient's daughter as it could lead to physical confrontation or worse. In addition, there may be more to this situation than meets the eye. Perhaps, the daughter is responsible for the patient's care and has an advance directive to feed the patient that may not be specified on the sign in the front of the room. You just don't know.

Second, you may want to reflect and say something like, "Sorry... I see you are upset. Why don't I leave the room and get you someone that may know more about the situation and can help you out." You can then temporarily step out of the room and recruit the help of the caring physician or the nurse around the corner.

Your role as a radiology resident is not the total care of the patient. It is to be the physician that ensures the patient can go for a procedure the next morning. Therefore, it is appropriate to let the caring physicians and nurses know what is happening so that if there is a potentially life-threatening emergency for the patient, it can be taken care of expeditiously. Do not argue with the patient as it can lead to a more active confrontation!

The Obtunded Patient

On interventional radiology rotations, this is a frequently encountered dilemma. You go upstairs to the floors and you begin to consent a patient. Suddenly, you realize as you are going through the motions that the patient doesn't understand a word that you are saying. What do you do???

First thing, check the charts. See if there is anything in the chart that confirms that the patient is not competent to make a decision. If not, what do you do? Make sure to think about whether or not the procedure/test is truly indicated emergently. The consent can certainly wait if it is not emergent. On the other hand, if the procedure is truly necessary, step out and ask the primary covering physician- What is the patient's situation? Has there been a recent change in mental status? Is the patient on medications that are preventing him/her from understanding/responding to the consent? If there is a temporary change in mental status, maybe there is a better time/place to consent the patient.

If the procedure is emergent and really needs to be completed first thing in the morning, then what is the next step? It is your responsibility to find the person responsible for the patient's care when he/she is obtunded so that you can consent the patient. You may find an advanced directive in the chart that gives clear instructions as to who is responsible for this patient's care. Or perhaps, the nurse or physician may know whom to contact in this event. In either case, make sure to contact the patient's responsible decision makers prior to getting consent. If you do a procedure and it has not been consented by a patient with mental faculties at the time, the consequences can be dire including the potential for legal action. Never sign off on a procedure for an obtunded patient without written consent from the responsible party!!!

Lessons To Be Learned About The Uncooperative Patient

The uncooperative patient is usually "uncooperative" for good reason. As radiology residents, we are often not privy to all the information that may lead to the patient's attitude or actions prior to or during a diagnostic or therapeutic radiology procedure. Also, remember that you are not alone in making decisions for the patient. Always get help from other clinicians when needed. And, never make assumptions about the patient without getting the facts straight. Not following these guidelines can lead to patient care disasters!!!

CHAPTER 28

Can I Be Sued As A Radiology Resident?

• • •

As RADIOLOGY MEDICAL SCHOOL APPLICANTS, radiology residents, and full-fledged radiologists, we all dread the possibility of a lawsuit when we begin to practice radiology. Very rarely discussed, however, is the possibility of being sued during radiology residency. The good news: it is very unusual! One article (1) stated that there were only 15 legal cases and 10 law review papers that addressed physicians in training and standards of care on 2 large legal databases. And, these cases were not necessarily radiology residency specific. The bad news: although a remote possibility, it has happened several times in the past. So, this makes for an interesting topic that is not frequently addressed but is certainly a possibility. In this article, I analyze a few different sources on the web and in the literature to understand what conditions need to be met in order for the radiology resident to be sued. More specifically, we will analyze what standards of care need to be breached. Also, we will go through several ways radiology residents can prevent lawsuits in the future.

THE GROUNDS FOR A LAWSUIT

In order for a lawsuit to be successful against any physician in general, three requirements need to be satisfied. According to a recent article in Diagnostic Imaging (2), these are a breach, causation, and damages. Breach implies that the physician did not satisfy the requirement of the standard of care. Causation implies that the breach of duty caused the malpractice. And, damages imply that there was significant harm produced by the event. In today's article, I am going to explicitly discuss the issue of the breach without a discussion of causation and damages because the concept of a breach is what makes a malpractice case performed by a resident different from a fully trained attending.

Due to the standard of care being different for a resident, the definition of breach for a resident involved in a malpractice event becomes a little more complicated. In fact, over time, the standards of what breach means for the radiology resident have become blurred. I will discuss several cases that have different definitions of what is considered to be "standard of care", specifically for a resident in training.

Some cases have involved the medical intern. There was one case when an intern failed to identify retained glass fragments and sewed a wound shut. In this case, it was concluded that the criteria for the standard of care should be based upon the standards for the typical skills of an intern at that level. Subsequent lawsuits have demonstrated that the first year resident needs to fail to do something that a "physician or surgeon of ordinary skill, care and diligence" would typically do in order to breach the standard of care rule. In other words, a first year resident without a full license can be required to meet the standards of a general practitioner physician in terms of standard of care.

For residents in a subspecialty level training program, there is added confusion related to the issue of breach of the standard of care. Some cases imply that the sub specialized resident should meet the requirements of a general practitioner and other cases imply that the resident should meet the requirements of a more specialized physician. Adding more confusion to the issue, according to the same article, there was one radiology resident specific case of a misread MRI of a newborn. In this case, the court was unable to determine a specific standard of care for the resident and ruled in favor the defendant. So, the "standard of care" for this radiology/specialist resident was not well defined at all in this case. (1)

In another case with a radiology resident, an AJR article (3) discussed an incident that occurred during radiology moonlighting. The resident was sued for missing an abscess and instead called it a bladder diverticulum on a CT scan. The lawsuit was eventually settled, but prior to the settlement, the court determined that the jury would determine the liability, implying that a standard of care was breached at the level of an attending subspecialist/radiologist.

So, according to the literature, sometimes residents are considered to have lower than the typical standard of care for attendings, other times they are considered to be at the level of the standard of care of a general practitioner, and at other times the resident has to meet the standard of the attending in his/her subspecialty. Confusing, huh?

What Does This All Mean? Primary Take-home Messages to Reduce Liability

So, now that you are really confused, what does this mean to you?

Precept 1: Regardless of the definition of breach for the radiology resident, make sure to get help if you are unsure and the case can lead to patient morbidity. This can reduce the odds of getting sued for a questionable interpretation and allows your fellow attending to take responsibility for the case.

Precept 2: If moonlighting, make sure you have malpractice insurance. Misses do happen and it is possible you may be treated as a fully trained radiologist. So, don't be caught off guard without proper insurance. In fact, you need to make sure that your insurance will specifically cover you for moonlighting mishaps.

Precept 3: Although it is infrequent, lawsuits do happen to radiology residents and you are certainly not immune from the ravages of the legal system. So, treat each case as if you are the responsible party and always provide your best effort to make the correct findings, diagnosis, and management.

Final Bottom Line

Although unlikely, residents can still be sued for malpractice. Don't leave yourself susceptible to the possibility of a lawsuit as a resident!

REFERENCES

(1) Clin Orthop Relat Res. 2012 May; 470(5): 1379–1385.
Published online 2012 Jan 26.
Medical Liability of the Physician in Training
Brian Wegman, MD, James P. Stannard, MD, and B. Sonny Bal, MD, JD, MBA corresponding author

(2) Radiologists, Expect to Get Sued March 03, 2016 | RSNA 2015, Practice Management By Liza Haar

(3) AJR1998;171:565 Malpractice Issues in Radiology: Liability of the Moonlighting Resident By Leonard Berlin

CHAPTER 29

Radiology Resident- Get Up And Move It!!!

● ● ●

SITTING CAN BE HAZARDOUS TO your health. Just take a look at some of the article headlines and links from major news organizations- <u>CNN</u> (1), <u>CBS</u> (2), <u>Huffington Post</u> (3). And, the list goes on...

What do we picture radiologists doing all day? Unfortunately, the stereotype is that radiologists are sitters; we are in a comfy chair near a diagnostic workstation, powering through loads of studies. There's some truth to that. In fact, I can almost guarantee that you will gain that freshman fifteen pounds during your first year of residency if you follow the typical work schedule without modifying your behavior. That's the bad news. The good news is that there are ways to circumvent the habit of sitting down for long periods of time, even as a radiologist.

And, since residents are early in their career, it is easier to start forming habits that will potentially last a lifetime. So, here are some suggestions to conquer the ills of long-term sitting, whether you are a radiology resident at work or at home.

1. STAND UP

Many desks these days allow you to complete your work while standing. In fact, we have several workstations dedicated to the standing radiologist in our own department, although unfortunately not enough.

But, let's say that this option is not available. What can you do to remind yourself to get up? I recommend either a watch timer or an Apple watch. Regularly, I get messages on my watch to tell me to stand up. It can be occasionally annoying, but it usually does the trick even though there are times I am unable to get out of my seat.

Additionally, little things help. Instead of texting your colleagues, consider getting up and having a conversation with someone. Instead of calling the technologist to complete a study, get up and tell them. These are ways you establish connections with people and lessen the amount of time you are sitting during the day.

2. GET THE MOST CALORIE BURN OUT OF YOUR WORKSPACE

Whenever I am at work, I always think about ways to maximize my body's workload. Think about calorie burning activities like banning the word elevator from your vocabulary. In fact, the only time I take the elevator is when there is a "wet paint" sign on the stairs. Using the stairs is a great way to burn those extra calories

Take a long way around to get to your next meeting or conference, whether it means going outside or visiting your colleagues. Just remember to leave your workstation a little bit earlier!

3. GET THAT HEART RATE UP- FIND A NEW ACTIVITY YOU CAN STICK WITH!

Any activity that doesn't interest me, I find difficult to stick with. And, I think it is easy to extrapolate the same for others. So, find something that increases your heart rate, but most importantly find an exercise routine that you enjoy. And, it is crucial to do so. Remember, radiologists sit down more than most other professions and you certainly don't want to add home sitting time to your total.

For instance, I started running several years ago and have continued diligently only because I look forward to the run. Why? It's very simple. I have my Ipad set up to watch <u>Netflix</u> (4) and <u>HBOGO</u> (5) shows that I find hard to watch without interruptions by just sitting down. Some of the series that I have gone through include Game of Thrones, The Sopranos, House of Cards, and Mad Men, among many others. So, I really look forward to my time on the treadmill.

Also, you may want to find activities that intrinsically interest you because you are learning something new, whether it is physical, mental, or practical. I have taken up Tae Kwon Do and have found it to be a great way to build up my stamina, flexibility, and coordination. Each lesson I take, I find that I am learning new things and want to come back for the next time.

The Bottom Line

Getting out there and moving is especially important as a radiologist because of the increased sedentary lifestyle and the years that you can potentially lose due it's health consequences. So, make a concerted effort to get up and move!!!

(1) http://www.cnn.com/2015/01/21/health/sitting-will-kill-you/

(2) http://newyork.cbslocal.com/2014/01/20/sitting-at-work-for-hours-can-be-as-unhealthy-as-smoking/

(3) http://www.huffingtonpost.com/the-active-times/sitting-is-the-new-smokin_b_5890006.html

(4) http://netflix.com

(5) https://play.hbogo/com/login

CHAPTER 30

Staying Healthy For Residency (And Life) (Leonard Morneau, MD)

● ● ●

*"The only insurance of your health are
the choices you make every day."*

– Leonard Morneau, MD

Residency is arguably one of the most grueling times of a physician's career/life. You're working long hours (80 hour weeks can be the norm), usually don't get enough sleep, and barely have time for yourself. At times, residents can get so focused on the health of their patients that they forget about their own health and well-being. This is a very sad turn of events. Physicians are supposed to be leaders in healthcare and it's my personal belief that the only way to lead is by example. Now you may be saying, but I don't have time to be healthy! I barely get enough sleep, there's no time for exercise! But the fact is that you can still be healthy even while working such strenuous hours. This is especially important for radiologists that spend most of the day sitting in a chair. The previous chapter does a great job explaining the importance of exercise and the different types you can do to stay active, even with minimal time. The main focus of this chapter will be on other healthy lifestyle choices to make.

The MOST important thing, by far, is the choice of what food you put into your body. I'll be honest; the cards are stacked against you here.

It's one of the main reasons we have the obesity epidemic and millions upon millions of people who suffer from completely preventable diseases. Our bodies have been engineered to desire sugar, fats, and other bad food choices. Why? Thousands of years ago when food was scarce it was good to have fats to store energy for later use in case of famine or not being able to find food. So the human brain was trained to crave those sorts of foods. Fast forward a few thousand years and those impulses are still here, but the food is plentiful (in most places).

In my personal opinion, most of the food choices we have today are very unhealthy. They're packed with sugar, preservatives, and other things that are simply not good for the human body. Yet this is the majority of food that's produced, is heavily advertised, and can be as addictive as a drug. Multiple studies have shown these addictive properties and that sugar specifically activates the same receptors in the brain as cocaine and heroin... (1,2,3) This is why "dieting" is so hard; it's like trying to tell someone addicted to drugs that they need to stop. Easier said than done.

INSTEAD, what must be done is not to think of things in terms of this diet or that diet, but living a healthy LIFESTYLE. There is no magic pill. It is the choices you make every day. Now, here's a list of some things you can do to start living healthier:

1) WATER

I recommend only drinking water (preferably hydrogen enriched water). Nearly all beverages are loaded with sugar, so ALWAYS check the nutrition facts. I've seen a "green juice" marketed to be healthy with "no sugar added" that contained almost 40g of sugar... And sugar is immediately converted to fat if it's not utilized by the body (which is most of the time, unless you just finished a tough workout). This is one of the easiest things you can do that will drastically improve your health. A good starting point is ½ your body weight in ounces of water daily.

2) EAT MORE GREENS

No one ever got obese by eating too many vegetables. Vegetables are nutrient dense foods (high in nutrients and low in calories) and they fill you up faster. For those of you complaining about them not tasting good enough for you, there's a ton of different ways to prepare veggies that taste amazing. I do it every week in my meal prep. Also, growing more plants for food consumption would be better for the environment and help slow the pace of global warming as well.

3) AVOID THE AISLES

When you go to the grocery store, the majority of your food should be purchased from the periphery of the store. Most of the food in the aisles of a typical grocery store is all processed, full of sugar and bad for you. Always check the nutrition facts before you buy something, you'll be amazed at what you're actually eating.

4) PREP FOR SUCCESS

Take one day a week to prepare most of your meals, at least lunch. This way you'll have healthy meal choices ready during the week. I've been doing it for years and it is definitely one of the main reasons I've been able to stay so healthy.

5) AVOID FAST FOOD

Restaurants like McDonald's, Burger King, Wendy's, etc. should be avoided like the plague. Compare eating fast food to using drugs like cocaine and heroin in your mind (after all they have a similar effect) and you'll be less likely to eat them. (I haven't been to one in nearly 4 years, so yes, it's possible).

6) Have A Cheat Day

With all the new changes to your diet, you're likely to crave those old foods that you love. Try to save them for one day of the week only. This will make it easier to eat healthier during the week when you know you have a reward coming at the end of the week. The less you consume these food choices, the less you will crave them.

7) Track It

Many people find that they're not aware of how much they're eating until they make a note of it and calculate out how many calories they take in. Try using an app just one day a week to see how much you consume in a typical day. It may be the eye-opener you need to kick-start a new lifestyle.

8) Snack Healthy

Instead of going for that cookie or other sweet in the mid-morning or afternoon, try having a healthier option like a handful of almonds or nuts.

9) Keep A Balance

Think of health as a bank account. Every good health decision you make, like eating vegetables and exercising, is a deposit. Every time you eat unhealthily or make such decisions you are making a withdrawal. Keep a tally of your deposits and withdrawals like you would your bank account. Just like it takes time to build wealth, good health is only obtained from making these deposits every day. If you withdraw more than you deposit, you'll go into debt and suffer the consequences. How does your account balance look?

It may seem difficult at first, but the habits you form today determine who you will be tomorrow. Keep the end goal in mind and you'll be able to do more than you ever thought imaginable.

Just as in airplane safety videos, they always tell you to put your oxygen mask on before your children's mask; Why? Because you're no help to that child if you're dead. Similarly, we must make our own health our first priority because, without it, we won't be able to take care of others; which is the whole reason we got into this profession in the first place.

(1). Spangler, Rudolph, Knut Wittkowski, and Noel Goddard. Opiate-like Effects of Sugar on Gene Expression in Reward Areas of the Rat Brain. N.p., 19 May 2004. Web. 14 Nov. 2016.
http://www.sciencedirect.com/science/article/pii/S0169328X04000890

(2). Colantuoni, C., J. Chwenker, and J. McCarthy. "Excessive Sugar Intake Alters Binding to Dopamine and Mu-opiod receptors in the brain : NeuroReport." LWW. N.p., 16 Nov. 2001. Web. 14 Nov. 2016.
http://journals.lww.com/neuroreport/Abstract/2001/11160/Excessive_sugar_intake_alters_binding_to_dopamine.35.aspx

(3). Avena, Nicole, Pedro Rada, and Bartley Hoebel. Evidence for Sugar Addiction: Behavioral and Neurochemical Effects of Intermittent, Excessive Sugar Intake. Neuroscience & Biobehavioral Reviews, 2008. Web. 14 Nov. 2016.
http://www.sciencedirect.com/science/article/pii/S0149763407000589

Section 3: Radiology Career Advice

● ● ●

CHAPTER 31

How To Choose A Radiology Fellowship

● ● ●

For some people, choosing a radiology fellowship is easy. They may have known they wanted to be an interventional radiologist or pediatric radiologist since they were 2 years old. But, for the majority of us, it is a more challenging decision. And, it is a decision that cannot be taken lightly. It has a direct effect on the type of practice (generalist or specialist), your lifestyle (academic vs. private practice), location (rural vs. urban), the types of people that you will see on a daily basis (direct patient care vs. indirect patient care), and more! So, I have come up with some guidelines for making this agonizing choice. Some of this decision should be based on your personality, what kind of lifestyle you want, the desire to make a little bit more money, the need to be in a certain location, application competitiveness, and gamesmanship/trends in the different subspecialties. I am going to divide the radiology fellowship decision tree into these six parts and describe how you should utilize each factor in order to choose your future subspecialty area. Let's start with the first factor...

Personality:

You can't deny who you are and you can't let others make that decision for you. If you hate working with your hands, interventional radiology is not going to be for you, regardless of your attendings' opinion of your performance. And, it behooves you not to decide to enter the field because you will be doing what you hate. Likewise, if you can't stand being near patients, mammography is certainly not an appropriate specialty, even if you are great with people. When you take your personality type into consideration, you've already significantly limited the playing field. I am going to list several personality types and make a list of the appropriate possible specialties for you. Your own personality type may differ from the one's listed below. If that is the case, you should think about your own personality type and come up with a different cluster of several different fellowship options.

Gregarious and outgoing- General Radiology, Interventional Radiology, Mammography, Pediatric Radiology

Fiercely independent- General Radiology, Interventional Radiology, and Neuroradiology

Introvert- Body Imaging, MSK Radiology, MRI, Trauma and Emergency Radiology

Jack of all trades- Body Imaging, MRI, Nuclear Medicine

Likes working with hands/interventions- Body Fellowship, Interventional Radiology, Mammography/Women's Imaging

Nurturing and friendly- Mammography/Women's Imaging, Pediatric Radiology

Techie- Body MRI, Informatics, Interventional Radiology, Neuroradiology (Interventional and Nonintervention), Nuclear Medicine

And so on and so forth...

LIFESTYLE:

So, you've decided upon your personality type... Next issue is what kind of lifestyle do you want. When I mean lifestyle, I am thinking about the following factors. Do you want to be academic or nonacademic? Do you want to become the "go-to-guy" for your specialty because you know a specific subspecialty in depth? Do you mind being on call late at night? Do you want to be in a small or large practice? So let's go through each fellowship option and determine the lifestyle factors of each of these subspecialties. Add these factors to the personality factors in order to hone your choice of subspecialty further.

Body Imaging/MRI- Most often practices general radiology without mastery of a single subspecialty area, Allows for academic and nonacademic possibilities, Can practice in a very small or large practice

Cardiothoracic Imaging- Most often practices in his/her subspecialty in an academic and large practice, Master of single subspecialty

Informatics- Needs to work in a large or academic center, Allows for increased possibility of entry into the business domain, Master of individual subspecialty

Interventional Radiology- Allows for practice of general radiology or mastery of individual subspecialty, Allows for small or large practice, Can be clinical or academic, Tendency for long call hours

Musculoskeletal Imaging- Allows for practice of general radiology or mastery of individual subspecialty, Allows for small or large practice, Can be clinical or academic

Neurointerventional Radiology- Most often practices in his/her subspecialty in an academic and large practice, Master of single subspecialty, Tendency for long call hours

Neuroradiology- Can work in large or small practice, Can be academic or nonacademic, Master of individual subspecialty

Nuclear Medicine- Tendency to be situated in a larger practice, Can be academic or nonacademic, Most often is a generalist

Pediatric Radiology- More often academic or related to a large practice, may be more predisposed to night time calls (i.e. intussusception reductions), Master of a subspecialty

Trauma/ER radiology- Most often in a large or academic practice, most often a generalist, Tendency toward nighttime work

Women's Imaging/Mammography- More options for part time hours and less call, Can be academic or clinical, Can be in a small or large practice, Master of individual subspecialty and less likely to be a generalist.

MONEY:

Fortunately, you've entered the world of radiology and all of its subspecialties within the United States tend to be higher paying than most other specialties. And, the distribution of salaries (1) is fairly equal among all subspecialties. However, there is a slight discrepancy/increased income in the interventional-based subspecialties such as Interventional Radiology and Neurointerventional Radiology, mostly based on the amount of time working rather than bringing in more income. Money should, therefore, play a minor role in the decision tree.

LOCATION:

Location can be an important factor in choosing a fellowship subspecialty because some fellowships may limit you to larger cities and/or academic centers. Take this into consideration if you need to be in a more rural locale for family reasons, etc. Remember this issue if you want to practice in the more academic subspecialties of Cardiothoracic Imaging, Informatics, Interventional Neuroradiology, Nuclear Medicine, Pediatric Radiology, or Trauma/ER radiology. This can potentially whittle down your choice of subspecialty further.

APPLICATION COMPETITIVENESS:

Competitive subspecialties cycle frequently over the years. For example, when I was a resident considering fellowship in 2002, you couldn't find anyone to enter the subspecialty of interventional radiology. Programs were desperate and would take anyone that graduated. Meanwhile, in 2014, the same specialty became an ultra-competitive fellowship and our residents had to send out numerous applications for the same spot. Therefore, if you have not performed well during your residency program or you come from a smaller program, you may have some difficulties entering a fellowship in some of the more competitive areas. Do not despair though. Most of the time, you can get into one of these more competitive areas. You just need to send out more applications and use your connections to your residency program.

Based on my recent experiences, some of the more competitive subspecialties in 2015 and 2016 include MSK Imaging and Interventional Radiology. But of course, that can change in any given year. You should still try to get into the more competitive specialties if that is what you desire. Just have a backup plan.

TRENDS/COUNTERTRENDS:

OK. So you've gone through the first 5 deciding factors and you probably have whittled down your choice substantially, but you're still not sure. There is still one more thing that you should probably consider before making your final decision. Currently, there are two secular areas of significant growth within radiology: big data/data processing and increasing applications of MRI.

So, consider this. You are probably better off picking an area of growth than one that may be more cyclical and subjected to the vicissitudes of the economic cycle. It's simply job security. Informatics and the MRI-based specialties certainly meet these criteria.

Also, I have found over the recent history of radiology, you are better off going against the grain, just like a contrarian investor in the stock market. You may consider in 1996 when Bill Clinton was talking about the socialization of health care and health care capitation, radiology became extremely unpopular. Those same residents that applied to radiology around that time had an unbelievable choice of places to work and could command their own salaries at the highest rate and work in the most desirable locations when they graduated in 2001-2003. On the other hand, when radiology was extremely popular in the mid-2000s lots of really strong applicants applied for radiology. Those same residents graduated in 2009-2012 and were very limited in their job prospects. The same situation will likely hold true for many of the less popular subspecialties at the current time. Take the contrarian view under consideration as well.

SUMMARY STATEMENT:

Using these criteria, you should certainly be able to narrow down your choice of subspecialties to one or two different possibilities at the most. Good luck with your final choice!

(1) http://www.auntminnie.com/index.aspx?sec=sup&sub=imc&pag=dis&ItemID=103466#nav-right

CHAPTER 32

The Informatics Fellowship- Bulletproof Your Radiological Future

● ● ●

CONCERNED ABOUT ARTIFICIAL INTELLIGENCE TAKING over our jobs? Worried about the economic cyclicality of each of the radiological sub-specialties? Do you fear the instability of your future radiology attending career due to corporate takeovers and mergers? Well, I have a solution for you (and no, I am not an infomercial!!!)... Welcome to the new fellowship called Informatics!!!

Why am I writing about the informatics <u>fellowship</u> (1) and skipping all the other subspecialties? Well... the informatics fellowship warrants an independent chapter because it is truly the only radiology subspecialty that is in a permanent secular growth trend. It is also the only fellowship that has relatively little information published on the subject matter. In fact, once several of my residents and students heard about the existence of the fellowship program and understood its potential benefits, they began to salivate!!!

So, this article is dedicated to the topic of the informatics fellowship. Specifically, we will discuss the definition of informatics, what the fellowship entails, requirements for the fellowship, how to find where to complete the fellowship, and what job opportunities are available for graduates of these programs. I think once you understand the potential benefits of this fellowship program, you might consider it yourself!!!

Discussion of Definition and Importance of Informatics

So, what is the definition of informatics? (2) According to Merriam-Webster, it is as follows- "the collection, classification, storage, retrieval, and dissemination of recorded knowledge". Prior to several years ago, I have to admit that I had never heard of the term or definition of informatics. In fact, I think I am probably not alone. It is only since the terms "the cloud" and "big data" have arrived into the mainstream that I think the word informatics has been used more widely.

Why is all of a sudden this body of knowledge so important? In our age of electronic interconnectedness, large swaths of data are created and processed every day. Particularly in the radiology realm, there are numerous electronic/digital images and reams of clinical/health information. Someone has to both understand and manage all this information. Although computer engineers presently manage a lot of this information, they tend not to understand how to manage the data for physicians, administrators, and patients to understand. Herein lies the niche of the radiology informaticist, translating the imaging and clinical data from the computer engineer to the clinical realm.

What Do These Informatics Fellowships Teach?

Fortuitously, the same day that I started to write about informatics, I received a letter from the APDR explaining that there would be a new initiative to create a summary online 1-week course in informatics for residents. Some of the topics covered by the course as listed in the letter include Standards; Computers and Networking; PACS and Archives; Security; Life Cycle of a Radiology Exam, Data and Data Plumbing; Algorithms for Image and Nonimage Analytics; and the Business of Informatics. This course contained many of the topics that some informatics fellowship programs teach. But, the curricula of many of the informatics fellowships differed significantly from this course and were more expansive.

To add a bit more confusion, each individual fellowship program also covers differing topics from one another and varies the emphasis of each of these subjects. Some of the topics that these fellowships include: RIS systems, Image Compression, Teleradiology, Quality Improvement, Operations, Clinical Engineering, HL7, Regulations, DICOM, Critical Results Reporting, Decision Support Systems, Radiation Dose Tracking, Mobile Health Applications, Image Segmentation, Imaging Room Ergonomics, 3D Printing, Natural Language Processing, Informatics Funding, Biostatistics, Health Policy, and Experimental Design. There was some overlap between the different programs. But coverage varied widely. I will also refer you to the ACGME formal program requirements in Clinical Informatics (3) for a more formal explanation of all the areas of teaching required at all fellowships.

What Are the Requirements To Become An Informatics Fellow?

The prerequisites vary from program to program. Of the programs I visited on the web, most but not all, had a requirement to be board eligible in a specialty (not necessarily radiology), to be a graduate of an American Medical School, and to have an interest in the discipline of informatics. Most fellowships did not have a specific requirement for formal training in computer science. According to the ACGME, the program length was 1 or 2 years to graduate from a radiology program.

Where to Find the Fellowships?

I found several ways to find the informatics fellowships that are offered for diagnostic radiology program graduates. If you happen to be a member of the AMA, you can look up the fellowships on the FREIDA database. (4) (It turns out I am not a member!) Alternatively, you can do a web search on informatics fellowships and many of the large institutions describe their own programs. And finally, you can go to the ACGME website (5) and look up informatics fellowships there.

Job Opportunities for the Informatics Fellowship Graduate

This is where things get really interesting... Job opportunities are endless. You want to be part of a large private practice or maybe a teleradiology practice? Interested in becoming a practice leader? It's all yours! Not many employers can replace the only radiologist that can fix a PACS or RIS system and can also actually read films.

Do you want to become an entrepreneur and start your own company? You will have access to all the tools and methods to create a technological niche for yourself whether it is an app, a PACS add-on, a new piece of software, or other countless unimaginable outlets.

Do you want to go into academics? The world is yours. Academics are desperate to have radiologists translate their IT department workings into something that is useful and efficient for clinicians. Think about the possibility of chairman or CIO.

Do you want to work for big business? Think Apple, Google, Cerner, and more! Large organizations are constantly on the lookout for good talent that can translate the engineering esoteric data into clinical reality. You will be able to develop needed applications, improve health and radiology related products to get more clientele, and more:

Think about it... you will be at the forefront and crossroads of technology and clinical medicine- a job that only a few can currently fill. It will be very difficult to replace you.

Diagnostic readers can be outsourced to India. Robotics can replace human procedures. But humans will always be needed to rule the machines (unless our future is to be the same as The Terminator!) (6)

Final Thoughts

Of course in the end, like anything else, you need to like what you are doing in order to be good at it. And, informatics is certainly not for everyone. But, if you have a remote interest in the intersection of computers and radiology, really consider this subspecialty. The possibilities are endless, job opportunities abound, and you have the ability to be in charge of your own destiny, potentially not subject to the whims of government or even private industry. You can be your own captain!!!

(1) http://radsresident.com/2016/10/09/how-to-choose-a-radiology-fellowship/

(2) https://www.merriam-webster.com/dictionary/informatics

(3) http://www.acgme.org/portals/0/pfassets/programrequirements/381_clinical_informatics_2016.pdf

(4) https://www.ama-assn.org/life-career/search-ama-residency-fellowship-database

(5) https://apps.acgme.org/ads/public/reports/report/1

(6) https://en.wikipedia.org/wiki/The_Terminator

Radiology Private Practice Versus Other Career Pathways- Is It Worth "The Extra Money"?

• • •

THE HERCULEAN QUESTION UP FOR debate: is a private practice career path worth the extra money? In order to really answer this question, you have to know your standard career options. If you are talking about standard career options for the radiologist (not the alternative career paths (1) discussed in a later chapter), you can really divide it into three main choices: private practice, academic/government, and the hybrid model. Lucky for you, if you are reading this article and you are in the process of making this decision, you have come to right place. I have worked in the world of academics as a fellow, worked in the world of private practice at my first job out of training at Princeton Radiology, and presently work at Saint Barnabas Medical Center where we operate with a hybrid model (I was also formerly a resident at a program with a hybrid model-Brown University). So, I am uniquely qualified to talk about how to decide between each option and I am going to do just that!!! (Don't let other posers fool you!)

What is the difference in income for an academic practice radiologist versus a private practice radiologist? If you look at the Medscape Radiologist Compensation Report from 2016 (2), the academic radiologist made on average 262,000 dollars (in this category also is included the military and government physician). On the other hand, some of the other private practice type radiologists made significantly higher amounts: the office based solo practitioner- 434,000 dollars; the office based single specialty group practitioner - 386,000 dollars; and the typical hospital compensated radiologist- 381,000 dollars. So, if you take these debatable inaccurate academic and private practice numbers into account, then there is a pretty substantial difference between the income of a private practice and academic radiologist (almost 100-150 thousand dollars per year). But not so fast! In terms of numbers alone, the true compensation may not really account for other benefits like pension and health care. Employees that work for the government or large institution academic hospitals can sometimes get substantial fringe benefits such as a pension of 70-80 percent of the final salary, incredible health care insurance that you cannot get elsewhere, or other interesting perks such as free tuition for children in college. These are perks generally not available for the typical radiology private practitioner. If you take the pension alone, that could amount to a guaranteed (0.8)(262,000 dollars per year) or about 210,000 for the rest of your life based on 2016 salary numbers. In fact, you would need to have 5.24 million dollars in the bank to have that kind of money guaranteed on an annual basis assuming a 4 percent fairly risk-free return. So, the difference may not be as substantial as initially assumed upon first glance.

Now that I have debunked some of the income-based differences (there are always exceptions to every rule!), let's talk about the different models and help you to decide which option is the right one for you. Let's start!

THE ACADEMIC/GOVERNMENT MODEL

In the pure academic or government model, the primary goal is not reading films and making money. Instead, it is to publish, teach, or subsist (if you are talking about a place like the VA hospital!). Prestige and promotion are results of these activities. For comparison, the typical private practitioner couldn't give a lick about these job requirements. The philosophy is often: publish or perish!

The typical academic sort writes a lot, is always obtaining grants, and is heavily responsible for the teaching and welfare of his/her residents. He/she typically reads fewer studies and sees fewer patients than a typical private practice radiologist. But, that may vary depending upon the `institution for which you work. He/she gives many conferences, travels all over the country or the world to give lectures, mingles with other academic sorts on all different types of committees, and plays a big role in directing the future of radiology. Many of these radiologists have outside ventures and partnerships with different companies and academic centers since they are not entirely occupied with the standard day-to-day role of reading films. Some of the partnerships may be based on their research or area of expertise.

The higher-up academic radiologists manage their staff as chairmen and may be responsible for budgeting and hiring and firing depending upon the institution. Again, your mileage may vary depending upon the role that you have in the institution. This is all to say that your day-to-day work is somewhat less controlled by the almighty dollar. (Although many would say it still plays a nice sized role!)

THE PURE PRIVATE PRACTICE MODEL

What is private practice about? In general, it is about maximizing income and the numbers of patients that go through your system. Of course, there is also an element of quality. But the quality is there, to increase profitability. The almighty dollar tends to rule the day and all roads lead back to the almighty dollar. Employees and owners grind out films on a daily basis, day in day out. The philosophy: if you are not working, you are not making money.

Now, of course, it is essential that the private practitioner accomplishes other activities in the process of trying to make money. These folks may be responsible for some or all of the following practice needs: advertising, buying and selling equipment, strategic partnerships, mergers, maintaining relationships with hospitals, hiring and firing an army of numerous employees (possibly radiologists, technologists, janitors, nurses, physicists, and so on), maintaining and purchasing real estate, payroll, billing, legal issues, parking, and utilities. Academic hospitals/facilities typically take care of some or all of these issues in a typical academic/governmental practice. Therefore, you really need to enjoy playing many different hats and roles as well as being a self-motivated entrepreneur.

The Hybrid Private Practice/Academic Model

This is my current role. I like to think that I get the best of both the private practice and academic world. (Although some would like to say that is the worst!) The philosophy of the hybrid practitioner: A dabbler who likes to do some of the elements of both private practice and academia, but not in such depth.

So, how does the hybrid model work? First of all, there are a few variations on a theme. In my situation, I am involved in a hospital based private practice with a residency program and multiple covered hospitals and imaging centers. Others may be employed by a hospital but may be more tied to the private practice world via output bonuses and so on. But, essentially you are expected to teach, do a little bit of research, and also maximize your work output and thereby income by grinding through studies. Most of these practices are not involved in the purely academic activities such as obtaining grants. And, you will probably not be involved in typical pure private practice issues such as maintaining the building utilities.

The hybrid practitioner/dabbler likes to do a little bit of everything without having to delve into some of the serious academic and pure private practice issues. I was never interested in writing and obtain grants, but I certainly wanted to teach. I was not interested in dealing with some of the very basic issues of private practice, such as hiring/firing technologists, but yet I was interested in the mechanics of business and private practice. For the sort of person that likes to be a bit more generalist, the hybrid model is a great career path.

How To Make The Final Choice?

I think the final choice becomes a personality based thought process, not one that should be based on the different income constructions of each career model. If you hate business in all forms, work for the government or academia. If you hate writing and teaching, a private practice may be for you. And, if you love doing a little bit of everything, think about the hybrid model. Bottom line: You need to be true to yourself. Do what you like, not what others think you will enjoy. If you follow these precepts, you will make a great choice and have a fantastic career!

(1) http://radsresident.com/2016/10/30/alternative-careers-and-supplemental-income-for-the-radiologist/

(2) http://www.medscape.com/features/slideshow/compensation/2016/radiology

CHAPTER 34

My First Real Radiology Job- Do I Want Partnership?

• • •

EVERY ONCE IN A WHILE a resident or fellow will ask me "Should I take a partnership track versus a nonpartnership track position?" Or, "What questions should I ask about partnership when I interview for a job?" These can be some fairly difficult questions to answer since there are so many variables involved. I will tackle some of these issues here. I will also answer some common questions and clarify some misconceptions.

In order to make this chapter somewhat structured, I am first going to talk about the features of employed positions and ownership/partnership track positions, determine whether it makes sense to be a permanent employee or on a partnership track, and then I will elaborate on the questions that you should ask if you are fortunate (or unfortunate) to be placed on a partnership track. So, let's begin...

TO BE OR NOT TO BE-- A PARTNER!!!

What are the initial differences among jobs that are permanent employee versus partnership track positions? First of all, there are no hard and fast rules because some employee positions have features of partnerships and some partnerships have characteristics of employed positions. For the sake of simplicity, I am going to ignore these nuances and I am going to talk about the general features of each type of employment situation. You can further determine how the different features of your particular job offer apply to you.

Employed Positions

To start, most employees are paid a fixed salary that makes up the majority of their income. Some employees also may get a production bonus of some sort, but it tends to be a small percentage of the salary. Starting salaries of employed positions tend to be higher than partnership track positions at the beginning. But, they remain more stable or gradually drift higher for many years to come. If the partnership or practice is having a "banner" year, you will likely still get the same negotiated salary regardless of its profitability in most practices.

They also tend to be at the mercy of the employing body, whether it be a hospital system, partnership, or corporate entity. In general, employees tend to have less control over their situation. Their employers make business decisions. If you don't like the technologist, nurse, or administrator in your practice, you will still have to live with that person. You will not be able to change your PACS system. You may or may not be able to set your protocols. Bottom line. You are at the whim of your employers.

Also, in general, employed positions usually have particular sets of responsibilities written in the contract. If there is a responsibility that you perform that lies outside the realm of your negotiated contract, it is not required to accomplish that task unless your employer pays you for it. Being an employee, allows you to concentrate on radiology without having to deal with the day-to-day issues of running a practice. For instance, you don't have to worry about hiring, firing, buying magnets, billing, capitalizing on radiology trends, attending hospital events, and more. There is a lot that goes into the management of a practice that is not related to the direct practice of radiology and as an employee, you will likely be a lot less responsible for these activities. But everything comes with a price. You are selling your ability to control the entity you are working for.

And most importantly for some, employees are treated very differently when there are major practice changes. In today's rapidly changing practice environment, groups are merging; hospitals are buying out imaging centers; large corporations are taking over smaller entities. When a major event such as this occurs, the employee usually does not stand to benefit, as the employer of the practice will. Typically, when a practice is "bought out", the partners or employers will get a large sum of money to pay for the accounts receivable, equipment, real estate, goodwill, and so on/so forth. On the other hand, the employee will typically get nothing. Or even worse, the employee will be the first to be fired if there is a restructuring of the business.

PARTNERSHIP TRACK POSITIONS

Partnership track positions are usually paid a lower amount at the beginning than an employed position until you make "partner". There can be a substantial difference in the income that a partnership track employee makes versus a permanent employee. Many starting radiologists do not understand this concept, but it makes a lot of sense. You are paying for the equity/ownership of the partnership in two ways.

First, there is a concept called "sweat equity". "Sweat equity" is essentially a time commitment toward the partnership. This process can last almost any time interval. Most practices have a partnership track period that can last anywhere from almost immediately (in the early 2000s I knew of one fellow that was offered an immediate partnership prior to finishing fellowship!) to 10 years. Time to partnership varies depending on multiple factors. These include first and foremost, location. The more desirable the location, the more competitive the partnership position. And, the more years to partner the partnership track radiologist will be charged. Additionally, the time to partnership can be longer if you own equipment, real estate, and other assets. That makes sense because, in order to pay for that share in the partnership, you need to put in more "sweat equity". Time to a partnership is also affected by market conditions. If there are numerous radiologists looking for partnership positions, the practice will charge a longer period of "sweat equity" because of the high demand for a position and willingness of the partnership track position "to pay" for it.

Second, many practices expect the partnership track employees to buy-in monetarily to the practice at the end of the partnership track term.

This buy-in may be related to the accounts receivable and/or the owned assets of the practice. Buy-ins can range from a nominal amount to over a million dollars depending upon the assets owned. The buy-in can be paid for directly, by a loan, or by increased "sweat equity". This can be a very important factor in a decision to select a partnership track position.

Partnership track employees are also expected to be involved in practice building. You will not just be performing your daily duties as a radiologist, but you will be assisting and learning to accomplish other tasks outside of the normal radiologist purview. You may be involved with hospital committees, giving grand rounds, attending events outside normal business hours, and other important "non-radiologist" functions. These events are essential training for the partnership track radiologist to learn the business roles of the partner.

One thing that is important for the applicant to remember: No practice partner ever wants to create a partnership position just to get another partner!!! Partnership positions are only created by necessity. Why? It's pretty simple. It dilutes the equity of the preexisting partners (meaning that each partner will get a smaller share of the profits). There has to be a significant need to create a partner. These issues include lack of coverage in a particular subspecialty, need for more practice managers, etc. So, you need to remember that there is no such thing as an entitlement for a new partnership track position. You need to be prepared to work hard to gain a share of the partnership for that period of time.

WHAT ABOUT THE PARTNERS?

Partners of a practice are also usually paid a fixed salary but they earn a substantial portion of their income from the excess profits of the practice, usually a bonus. Usually, you expect the salary of the partner to be higher than that of the employee. Why? Partners assume the risk of the practice and also manage practice issues. If there is a decrease in reimbursement, partners are affected first. If there is a loss of an employee, the partner needs to cover that position. If there is a lawsuit against the practice, it is the responsibility of the partner to manage the issue. The difference in salary between a partner and a non-partner, however, can vary widely depending on the profitability of the practice. Therefore, it behooves the applicant radiologist to try to determine what the partners are making prior to joining the practice. You need to "check the books" or talk to the business manager. You certainly do not want to go through the process of "sweat equity", only to find out that your final income is not much different from your partnership track salary.

DOES IT MAKE SENSE TO BE ON A PARTNERSHIP TRACK?

Believe it or not, there is no quick answer to this question. It all depends on the individual situation and the job. There are also inherent risks to taking a partnership track position versus a permanently employed position. So, let's evaluate each piece of this equation individually with different questions.

Are you the sort of person that likes running the show or do you just want to do your work and go home?
A partnership track individual needs to be interested in business and practice building. There is no room for a partner that does not have any interests in building the practice outside normal business hours or is not willing to perform extra roles during the workday outside the normal radiology purview.

Is the job something temporary for you or do you want this job to be permanent?
You should not put "sweat equity" into a job when you think you will be leaving in several years to be closer to the family. You will be paid less for a partnership position that you will likely not have for more than a few years. It's just not worth it. Or maybe, you just need a position, but the practice job description is not exactly optimal and it is the only thing available in your desired location. In this case, you may also decide a partnership track is not the correct decision. For example, you don't want to

be practicing women's radiology when your only desire is to be an interventional radiologist!

What is the current business environment in the location that you are applying?
In some practice locations, private practice jobs are becoming converted
to employee positions due to mergers and acquisitions. You do not want to
be stuck on a partnership track, only to find out that there is no partnership position at the end of the road. You may never make the "partnership"
salary or even worse, you may be out of a job. Remember in a situation like
this- non-partners are the first to go.

Are there other issues like multiple recent retirees getting buyouts?
First of all, what is a buyout? It is essentially the opposite of the buy-in.
A partner that steps down expects to get the equity back that he put into
the practice. Every once in a while, a practice may have a large number
of former partners retiring with enormous buyouts. This can affect the
partners' salaries dramatically depending on the circumstances. You need
to look into all the specifics for yourself.

Is there a tiered partnership?
Some partnerships have separate buy-ins for the professional portion of
the practice and the technical ownership of the practice. Others may give
you only a small percentage of ownership compared to a "full partner". You
may become a partner one day. But, the partnership may not be what you
thought it would be. Some practices are "more equal" than others!!! It is very
important to get all the facts correct prior to starting that partnership track.

SHOULD STUDENT LOANS AFFECT THE DECISION TO BE ON A PARTNERSHIP TRACK?

I am going to try to tackle this question separately from all the others
because it is becoming an important issue for residents/fellows prior to
the partnership decision, given their large loan burdens. The difference

between an employed position and partnership track position can seem substantial at the beginning. And, it may or may not be more financially savvy to take the initial lower paying partnership track job. Here's where it is really important to try to glean the specifics of your prospective job. And, this decision can be complicated. You really have to plug in the numbers for yourself and make the calculations. To show you, we will take a specific circumstance under consideration. I will give you the example below.

Here are the inputs:

* You owe 500,000 dollars in student loans.
* Student loan interest and long-term investment returns are both 6%
* The partnership track lasts 3 years.
* The difference between the salary of a partner and an employee is 150,000 dollars.
* The permanent employee makes 100,000 dollars more per year on average than the partnership track position during the term of the partnership track.

Theoretically, the difference in salary can go to student loan payments if you are in a permanently employed position at the beginning. So, after taxes, you will have to say 66,000 dollars (100,000 dollars *0.66) per year or about 200,000 dollars (66,000 dollars x 3 years) more principal paid toward the student loans at the end of three years. Assuming the interest rate on the loan and the money you will make after you pay the loan is 6 percent, over the course of a 30-year career that same amount is equivalent to saving 200,000 *1.06^30 or approximately 1.15 million dollars.

On the other hand, if you decide to take the partnership track, you lost out on the 1.15 million dollars that you would have made if you were an employee. But, how much more, in the end, will you make to compensate for those years of "sweat equity"? So, let's take the difference in salary between a partner and a non-partner while taking the taxes out on a yearly basis. That number would be (150,000 dollars* 66 percent) or 100,000 dollars. Let's take that 100,000 dollars and multiply it by the number of years worked. That number would be 100,000 dollars *27 years (30 years of working minus 3 years of making less than an employee) or 2.7 million dollars. This number does not even include interest!! In this case, it would certainly make financial sense for the applicant to take a partnership track position.

The bottom line is that you need to perform the calculations for your own position. But, it may make financial sense to take the partnership track position even though the initial salary is less than the permanent employee.

Final Thoughts

The decision to become a partner in a practice vs. a permanent employee may not be simple due to the personality of the applicant, job-related factors, and monetary considerations. If you are thinking about the partnership route, make sure to know your role and get as much information/specifics as you can so you can make the leap. Becoming a partner is a long-term decision, just like a marriage. Know what you are getting into!!!!

CHAPTER 35

How To Combat A Difficult Radiology Job Market?

● ● ●

For several years, radiology has been slowly climbing out of a recessionary job market for its graduating residents. Although the market has been slightly improving, perhaps due to retiring senior radiologists and growth in imaging studies, the job market is still not wide open. And, many locations remain very competitive for new radiologists, especially on the east and west coasts. It is very difficult to find a partnership position in San Francisco or Manhattan!!!

So, how do you, as a graduating radiology resident or fellow, begin to approach finding a job in this competitive landscape? We are going to cover the essentials for finding a quality job in these difficult radiology markets. I will divide the essentials into the following sections: networking, diversification of skills, location, recommendations, and research/national organization involvement.

Networking, networking, networking!!!

Networking does not only begin when you start looking for a job. In fact, the search for the ideal job begins at home. What do I mean by that? Everything that you do as a radiology resident is monitored by your current attendings. And, the first and most important part of networking is maintaining good relationships with your colleagues and attendings.

Many attendings have their proverbial "ear to the ground" and can tell you about opportunities in the area. They can guide you to those jobs. In order to get access to these high-quality jobs, you need to perform and be a good team player. The resident that has not been "playing nicely in the sandbox" over the four years of residency and the final year or two of fellowship is not going to receive those insider tips. This resident is more likely going to have to fend for herself/himself. On the other hand, those residents that are constantly striving to become the best radiologist they can be and relate well to their colleagues will have first dibs on those desirable jobs when their attendings learn about them.

It also becomes more important than ever to stay in contact with your colleagues and coworkers. Even when you are ready to leave your residency to go to your fellowship, try to keep in touch with your former colleagues, whether it is your fellow residents or attendings. You never know when that next job lead is going to pop up. And, most of these people are going to be happy to give you a tip or two on any new leads as well as how to find that next great job.

What about social media? Nowadays, professional-based social media groups such as <u>LinkedIn</u> can play a role in getting that next job. It can be another means to keep in contact with your former colleagues and keep others aware of your current training and expertise. I think that most residents should maintain at least one account. But be careful to keep the account relevant and correct. View it like a resume. If it is not updated and contains false information, it can be a detriment toward finding that next great job. Otherwise, it can be a great way to contact your former colleagues and mentors as well as a way to get new leads.

Finally, even when you have started on that first job, whether it is a dream job or merely a stepping-stone, make sure to be cordial and appropriate to your interviewees. I remember when I was interviewing; I met with an attending at a practice that was touting the merits of his practice to me. I subsequently found a job with a different practice, different from his. However, 6 months later that same attending who interviewed me became an interviewee at my current practice. You never know what is going to happen!!!

DIVERSIFICATION OF SKILLS

As a resident and fellow, try to do things in your field slightly out of your comfort zone. What do I mean by that? You never know what practices are going to want. Things change. Sometimes practices may need a cardiothoracic radiologist but have a need for a radiologist that can also read mammography. Other times, a practice may need an interventionist that feels comfortable with reading musculoskeletal MRI. So, to become the most competitive candidate in your class, you need to make sure that you feel comfortable in as many modalities as is reasonable. The only way to do that is to not just concentrate on your fellowship skills or areas of comfort, but rather on your weaker procedures and modalities.

As a fellow, it also becomes crucial to moonlight to maintain your skills in other general radiology areas, different from your fellowship. It will build your speed and accuracy so that when you start your first job you will be able to read studies at a reasonable pace. This will allow you to have a greater likelihood of remaining at your first real job!

SHOULD LOCATION BE THE SACRIFICIAL LAMB?

Sometimes the job market in some locations may become so ultra competitive that it may not be possible to find a good job in your desired area. In that case, there are times when it makes sense to alter one's expectations and apply to other locales outside of one's original intentions. This may significantly increase the choices of the applicant and allow him/her to practice his/her own subspecialty or have a better income to support the family. This is a decision that should not be taken lightly, given that there may be personal or family issues. But, it is something that should be considered depending upon the living situation of the applicant/resident/fellow.

RECOMMENDATIONS

As a radiology resident or fellow, obtaining a recommendation for a radiology job is much different than asking for a recommendation as a medical student. Instead of a formal letter, typically a radiology resident or fellow will simply let the attending know to expect a phone call from a radiologist where he/she interviewed. The process is a bit more informal but is actually more informative than a simple letter of recommendation. It is easier to relay the true personality and information about a candidate on the phone than on paper. In the conversation, the caller may informally ask your attending of record what kind of resident you were and if you were a team player. Other times, a member of the practice may speak with a friend of theirs within your residency program to confirm that you would make a reasonable job candidate. Bottom line: It is good manners to let the attending you specify for a recommendation from your program to expect a phone call!

RESEARCH/NATIONAL ORGANIZATIONS

For those of you that may be interested in academics, staying involved in multiple research projects can be crucial to finding that first academic job. Although not as crucial for the private practitioner, it certainly can't hurt to also have good quality research under your belt when you look for that first job. As I've mentioned in the previous chapter called Tackling Research-Basic Issues And Considerations For The Radiology Resident, if there is a choice between two candidates that are equal, many times a practice may choose the resident with more research experience. You never know...

Also, getting involved in national organizations, whether it is the ACR, RSNA, or AUR, can be a great way to learn about the politics of radiology as well as to meet colleagues and practitioners. All residents should consider participation in these organizations, as it could be a stepping-stone to finding a great job or to become the next President!

FINAL THOUGHTS

If the job market is tough, all is not lost. Even in the toughest markets, there are usually a few jobs available. In order to increase your chances of getting one of these desirable slots, you may need to work a bit more intelligently and focused on becoming a desirable candidate. Networking, diversifying your skills, making sure to get great recommendations, finding the correct location, and participating in research and national organizations can help your cause. Ultimately, these practices will choose someone that fits the expected identity of an ideal candidate. If you follow these essentials, you have a much better chance that person will be you. Good luck!!!

CHAPTER 36

Alternative Careers And Supplemental Income For The Radiologist

● ● ●

EVERY ONCE IN A WHILE, a frustrated resident will say to me, "I'm not sure if I am interested in any of the traditional fellowships in radiology. What else can I do with my life? I am 250,000 dollars in debt and I don't think I can stomach practicing radiology like everyone else for the rest of my life. I have no choice." It is tough to think that after all the money, time, and effort, you have invested into a radiology residency, there may not be a career at the end of the road that you will enjoy. In addition, many radiologists think that if you are not practicing in one of the standard subspecialties, you are a waste to the specialty. And finally, many radiologists are not aware of all the opportunities out there in the world. But given these biases, it is no wonder this sort of atypical resident would need to address feelings of hopelessness.

Some radiologists and radiology residents just need other outlets for their talents and to find a different path. And, in truth, the potential for any radiology resident to have a career outside the confines of typical radiology practice that pays well and is intellectually rewarding is almost endless. Just remember, it is not an easy journey to get to the promised land of the alternative career opportunity. People that decide to take these alternative pathways may burn the proverbial "midnight oil" and take years to become an expert in an alternative career and become the top of their prospective field. But, if you are interested in seeking these possibilities, you have come to the right chapter!!!

Also, there are some radiologists that merely want to supplement their income from other sources in another area where they may have an interest. We will certainly discuss some of those possibilities as well.

So, I am first going to address where to look for these opportunities. And, in the second half, we will address the opportunities themselves, both the full-time career pathways and the supplemental income pathways.

Alternative Careers- Where to Look?

All physicians should know that there are outlets that exist for getting information and networking about alternative career opportunities. Let me give you a few that I know. First of all, there is a website out there that regularly posts jobs and career options outside of the mainstream radiology career path for physicians and healthcare professionals called the dropoutclub.org. This website posts all sorts of jobs that are currently available for physicians and contains a forum that discusses different issues for physicians seeking an alternative career. There are even sections within the website that approach how to interview for certain job types such as consulting.

There is also a website called seak.com that specializes in the area of legal/expert witness testimony. But, the website also contains information on all sorts of alternative career paths. In addition, there are loads of seminars and opportunities to potentially network with other physicians in a similar situation.

Some recruiters are actively involved in finding residents and attendings that have interests in other career opportunities. They can sometimes be a helpful resource and may know of available jobs that may be relevant to the physician's interests. But let the buyer beware! Although many recruiters are legitimate and truly want to help the physician, there are others that just want to make the sale at any cost even though the job or the career path may not be right for the applicant.

Finally, there may be physicians that you work with on a regular basis that perform other activities outside the daily practice of radiology. From my experience, I have encountered some colleagues that have started their own consulting business, invented medical devices, worked as an expert witness, wrote books, or performed other career activities outside of the typical realm of radiology. These people are great resources to learn about how to get a start in some of these alternative careers. I recommend talking to these people because they will give you a more realistic insight into traveling down these pathways that you may not get from a seminar, website, or recruiter.

WHAT ARE SOME OF THE OPPORTUNITIES?

In the interest of time and space, I cannot go into all the specifics of each career opportunity, but we can certainly paint some broad strokes about many of them. I will divide some of these opportunities into the following sub-segments- Finance, Legal, Political, Consulting/Surveys, Pharmaceutical Companies/Research, Invention/Entrepreneurial, Teaching, and Writing. There are certainly other areas as well, but these are some of the areas that are most familiar to me that I can comfortably talk about.

FINANCE

Let's start with finance, an area that lends itself to the alternative full-time career. This area seems to be one of the most "sexy" for many radiologists and radiology residents. You may think high pay, high profile. When you log on to the dropoutclub website (1), many of the posted jobs are in this realm. There are many hedge funds and large brokerage houses that seek people who can understand how companies operate in the biotechnology and medical world that may not be readily accessible to the typical layperson. Radiologists have a particular set of expertise in imaging devices and this focus may allow insight into companies that other medical professionals don't have. You may be involved in the tasks of research and presenting information to the executives of a company. Or you may be involved in gathering information from clinicians. Some of the positions are geared to the entry-level job and others are geared to the more experienced professional with finance experience. It is important to remember that you will probably be starting out low on the totem pole unless you have a strong finance background. Long hours are the norm. But, there is a very high pay potential. Just like becoming a full-fledged radiologist, it is a long road!!

LEGAL

Let's split this career pathway into two parts: becoming a litigator and expert witness work. The first pathway involves a full career change. You may hear of physicians that have also obtained their JD degrees to work in areas such as malpractice defense or even patent work. Both of these areas certainly lend themselves to the expertise of the radiology trainee. Getting a JD, may involve another 3 years of schooling with additional significant expense as well as a long path to a partner within a firm. So, this can be a tough road. Alternatively, you can think about doing this later on in your career after you have paid down some student loans. When there is a will there is a way!

More commonly, many radiologists participate in expert witness testimony as a way to supplement their income and maintain a footing in the legal realm. This pathway involves reviewing cases and providing opinions to attorneys. On occasion, you may even be involved in expert witness testimony or a deposition in court. Some physicians exclusively provide support for the defense of physicians and others may work for either side. It can certainly be interesting work and can give you a new perspective on the legal side of radiology and medicine.

POLITICAL

Ever thought about becoming the next <u>Ben Carson</u> (2) or <u>Bill Frist</u>? (3) If they can do it, you certainly can too. Some residents are politically inclined. They may like being involved in hospital committees and organizations.

They also may like being in charge of their residency program as chief resident and being involved in liaison work between the attendings and residents. If this is the avenue you want to take, there are certainly ways of making your future success more probable.

I would recommend residents to look into the <u>Rutherford-Lavanty Fellowship in Government Relations</u> (4), organized by the ACR. According to the website, "it allows residents to gain an understanding of state and federal legislative and regulatory processes and the ACR role therein. It also informs residents about the governmental factors that play important roles in shaping the future of radiology." This would be a perfect entree into the world of political action. There are also annual meetings such as an interesting <u>RLI Leadership Summit</u> (5) held annually where residents can learn about health care leadership opportunities.

I also think this sort of resident should get involved in hospital, regional, and/or national organizations and actively seek opportunities to participate in leadership roles. Half of politics is networking. The bigger your network, the more likely you can get involved in a political career.

Consulting

The word consulting is a very broad term. Consulting work incorporates many different entrepreneurial and employed entities as well as part-time work such as surveys. So, I am going to divide it into two parts.

Consulting as a career

I will begin with the full-time career path. There are some companies that specifically hire physicians to provide expert consultation for businesses. One such well-known company is called <u>Mckinsey & Company</u>. (6) In addition, there are niches in which someone with a unique background may have expertise. If you have prior training and interest in software engineering, for instance, you may want to utilize your skills to become an independent consultant in the area of software development, PACS, etc. You can potentially leverage this area of expertise to start your own company or work with large companies to assist in product development, increasing efficiency and customer satisfaction, and more. Consulting work is unique to the individual's talents, opportunities, and imagination.

Survey work

Many physicians, such as myself, will occasionally participate in telephone or Internet surveys. Often times, a consulting company will want to get the input from radiologist about new products or the business/political environment. There are a bunch of different companies to which you can sign up and get involved with their surveys. I make sure when I participate in these surveys that the time spent is worth my while. I have found the following survey/consulting companies to be fairly reliable, compensate fairly well, and have a decent amount of work for radiologists: GLG group (7) and M3 Global Research. (8) Be careful not to participate in surveys from companies that only offer prizes for a random winner without guaranteed compensation. It's probably not worth your while. You are a professional and your time is certainly worth something!

Pharmaceutical Companies/Research

There are many opportunities for physicians in this realm. Again, you will be starting at the very bottom. You just have to accept that. But, there have been some very interesting opportunities available for radiologists.

At my former job, I participated in the reading of imaging studies for pharmaceutical clinical trials. Many large companies still want physicians/radiologists reading their images to make their studies more powerful and legitimate. You can also get involved in structuring the studies and negotiating with companies to provide these services when you get to a higher level within the company.

Additionally, if you are inclined toward research, there are many opportunities to run a research department in a large pharmaceutical company, typically imaging research. Many pharmaceutical companies also give significant opportunities to radiologists/physicians to climb the corporate ladder. Remember though, there is certainly a bit less stability with a pharmaceutical company career, compared to the typical radiology career. But then again, you are reading this because you are not the typical radiologist!

Invention/Entrepreneurial

Maybe you have the next great idea. And, you just need an avenue to implement it. There are many radiologists who have gone down that pathway. Unfortunately, it does take a lot of work including research/development, funding, marketing/advertisement, salesmanship, and so on/so forth. There are also no guarantees that your product/idea is going to succeed. So, it is best to stick with your first career until the idea/product/company becomes large enough to support you full time. But, the rewards can be immense for the hard working entrepreneur.

Teaching

Many colleges and large universities need quality scientists to teach their courses. Radiologists certainly qualify!!! If interested in this realm, you may consider contacting a school to find out their needs. This can begin as a supplemental income or can become a career avenue. In addition, if you have a particular expertise in a certain area in radiology, there are also entrepreneurial opportunities to begin your own course/curriculum/school and build it over time.

Writing

Welcome to my world!!! I am fairly new to the blogging industry. But, it is a great way to get your name out there. In fact, starting a website and writing is a great platform for other career and business opportunities, whether it be writing a book, consulting, or whatever/wherever your interests lies. Also, if you have a hankering for this avenue, there are also many opportunities to write for others as a freelancer or work for medical organizations that need writers that can translate medical jargon to the general public. The opportunities are extensive. Of course, you can also decide to write the next great novel and become the next <u>Michael Crichton</u>!!! (9)

All These Pathways. So Little Time.

I bet many of you did not know that there were so many alternative careers pathways and avenues for supplemental income for the radiologist. So, for those of you that are not sure you want to stick with the typical radiology career, don't despair! All it takes is a bit of imagination, time, and hard work, and you too can find an outlet for your talents and your loves, whether it is a part-time gig or a full-blown career.

(1) https://www.dropoutclub.org

(2) https://en.wikipedia.org/wiki/Ben_Carson

(3) https://en.wikipedia.org/wiki/Bill_Frist

(4) https://www.acr.org/Advocacy/Rutherford-Fellowship

(5) http://www.radiologyleaders.org/meetings-and-courses/live-meetings/2016-rli-summit

(6) http://www.mckinsey.com/careers/search-jobs

(7) https://services.glgresearch.com

(8) https://www.m3globalresearch.com

(9) http://www.michaelcrichton.com

Appendix: Radiology Resident Financial Advice

• • •

APPENDIX A: PAYING BACK STUDENT LOANS VS. INCREASING SAVINGS- A DILEMMA!

• • •

CONGRATULATIONS!! YOU'VE FINISHED MEDICAL SCHOOL and you've collected your first few paychecks or perhaps you finally have a few extra dollars to spare. Feels good, huh.

But, you look at your monthly student loan statement, and you have debt ticking higher month after month. Perhaps it's not much, less than 100,000 dollars, or maybe it is 200,000, or even up to 500,000 dollars. Scheduled repayments may range anywhere from a few hundred dollars per month to multiple thousands of dollars with interest, of course. You feel a little queasy all of a sudden as you realize your predicament. What do you do?

Well, I've hiked up this mountain of debt already and have been fortunate enough to climb down. The good news is that someday you will too. The question is how and what is the best way to do it.

So, you finally may have your first job as a radiology resident and maybe you have an extra 100 or 200 dollars after your expenses for the first time. What do you do with the money? Do you pay down student loan debt or put it into a savings account/investments? That's an interesting question without a one size fits all answer. I will go through a rational method of making these decisions.

First off, we are assuming you have no high-interest credit card debt or other high-interest debt. That needs to be paid off first because you can never catch up your debts with interest rates over 10 percent. So, let's say that is the case, now some of what to do next depends upon the amount of student debt, your student loan interest rate, and your shorter term goals.

As a thought experiment, let's begin with what you may get back when you begin to pay off your student debt and you have a large amount taken out in student loans. At a resident salary level, you do get a <u>student interest tax</u> deduction (1) at the end of the year of up to 2,500 dollars on the interest serviced on the debt. So, if you have the money to pay off the student debt of 2,500 dollars and most or all of that goes back to interest (due to a large student loan), you will get back 15 percent assuming a salary of up to 65000-80,000 dollars in 2016 for a single person (deduction phases out between 65,000 and 80,000 dollars) and assuming a salary of up to 130,000-160,000 dollars for a married couple (deduction phase out between 130,000 and 160,000). Where can you make 15 percent interest on your money as a guarantee? Not many investments in this world will guarantee you that sort of return.

On the other hand, let's say you have a relatively low amount of student debt at a fairly low-interest rate. Most of the money that you pay back is going to go back to the principal and not the interest. Your return on investment is not going to be close to the 15 percent interest rate that you get back from the <u>student interest tax</u> deduction. (1) It will be closer to the true interest rate of the loan.

If you are fortunate enough to have a low-interest rate of up to 2,3, or 4 percent either by consolidating or refinancing your debt and you have small amounts of student debt, it makes sense to concern yourself more with the savings part of the equation. However, anyone with interest rates of over 4 percent, in today's low-interest rate environment, should really make loans their first priority. But in either case, low or high-interest student debt and small or large student loans, I always say diversify. What does that mean? Never put all your eggs in one basket. Put some towards savings and some toward student debt. Everybody needs some savings. Assess your interest rates and the amount of student debt to prioritize how much to dedicate to each bucket.

OK. Let's say now you are interested in saving for a larger emergency fund or maybe you need a down payment on a car or house. These may be necessities for your situation. Well, then you would want to take a fixed percentage of what you have left over at the end of the month and divide the total left over into two buckets. If your student loan interest rate is low and you have low amounts of debt, it would make sense to put a higher percentage of your leftover funds into the savings bucket (say 80 percent). And, if your interest rate and the amount of debt are higher, then you should probably consider putting less into saving (say up to 20-30 percent). This will allow you to build up your savings and to tackle your student loan debt.

This method will allow you to get control over your student loans over time while maximizing the amount of money saved for you and/or your family. And then, when the day comes that you get your first real job as an attending, you will appreciate the more manageable debt load and the savings that you have built up during your residency!

(1) https://www.irs.gov/publications/p970/ch04.html

APPENDIX B: SHOULD A RESIDENT PHYSICIAN APPLY FOR A CREDIT CARD WHEN ALREADY IN SIGNIFICANT DEBT?

● ● ●

CREDIT IS A VERY TOUCHY subject with resident physicians in all specialties lately. And, it makes sense. Student debt seems to be increasing exponentially over the years. When I graduated I thought I had a lot of debt from student loans. But in fact, that number pales in comparison to the amount of debt that most current medical residents hold. Confirming this suspicion, I did a miniature survey of almost 100 medical students at my current hospital. Student debt sums were as high as 600,000 dollars. And, these medical students had not even completed their four years of training yet. So, the amounts were even scheduled to be higher than that. These sums of money are not insignificant. But rather, the debt will be life altering for many of these future physicians. This all brings me to the next question. Does it really make sense for a resident to apply for a credit card after accruing so much debt? This question came up in the past year with a resident who had not started to get credit in his name. It caused all sorts of issues for him at the time it was needed. And, it will probably continue to cause issues for years to come until a good credit record is established. So, the simple answer is yes. But in this post, I will explain the reasons why establishing a few credit card accounts makes some sense even with significant debt. And, I will briefly discuss how residents should establish credit.

Why Do Resident Physicians Need A Credit Card?
Laying out Money

There are many times when a radiology resident needs to front a significant amount of funds for travel or other large purchases. What do you do if you do not have a credit card or do not have a credit card with enough credit? Nowadays, most travel is booked online with credit cards. For many websites, the only form of payment is the credit card. You are now stuck with either relying on others to book your flight or not going on the flight. Once you get to the level of a resident, these issues arise much more often.

Establishing a Track Record For Large Future Expenses (Mortgages, Car Loans, Etc.)

In order to purchase large items such as a house or a car without cash (and most residents don't have lots of cash on hand!!!), you need to obtain a mortgage or a loan. How is some company going to provide you with a loan if you do not have a long track record of making payments? Sure, you have your student loan as some background. But, that is not enough. You also have to have at least one revolving credit account (a credit card) in order to increase your credit score to obtain these large loans. A credit card is a great way of establishing this background.

Cash Back

Finally, many credit cards offer incentives in the form of airplane miles, gifts, and cash. I find that cash has the most value out of any of these rewards. When you make a purchase, you can get a certain amount refunded on every purchase. Some cards give you 5% on certain items or 2% on all items that you purchase. So, it really can add up over time. If credit is used wisely, it can really pay back dividends!

How To Establish Credit Without Breaking The Bank

If you have a poor or no credit history, it can be challenging to find a good credit card company willing to give you a credit card. Even with these issues, there are a couple of ways to establish credit. You can apply for cards that are backed by your own personal savings or find cards that have very low maximum balances. Either of these sorts of cards will allow you to make occasional small purchases so that you can begin to establish a credit history. And, remember to use personal credit hygiene: Pay your balances off entirely every month and try to use a small percentage of the credit allotted. These small steps will allow you to establish a good history without spending too much.

Summary

Even though resident physicians already have huge amounts of debt, establishing a credit card account becomes very important from both a practicality and utility standpoint. And, it can be done in a way that does not cause undue additional debt burdens or hardship. Bottom line: Make sure to establish credit now rather than later when you really need the credit!

APPENDIX C: I'M JUST A RESIDENT- SHOULD I REALLY START SAVING FOR RETIREMENT?

● ● ●

You've just started collecting your first few paychecks or you are a more seasoned 3rd or 4th-year resident. Either way, you may be thinking, I only have 50 dollars left over at the end of the month after paying off student loan interest, putting money into an emergency account, and paying off all my expenses. It's only 50 dollars- Does it really matter if I save it or spend it on dinner, drinks, and/or movies? Well, if you have that thought process month after month, you can be doing some serious damage to your future net worth. Let's run through some calculations.

The Basics of Compounding at Different Ages

So let's assume you are beginning residency and you are 26 years old. And let's say, you will also be working until you are 70 years old. That gives you somewhere around 45 years of a working life. Let's estimate that you can average 8 percent per year in your investments. (the stock market has given back close to 10 percent returns over the past century!) (1) So based on the 8% yearly return, your 50 dollars would be worth (50*1.08^45) or 1,596 dollars at the time of retirement. Of course, some of that money would be eroded by inflation. Now let's assume inflation is going to run 2.5%. That means that the 1,596 dollars would be eroded by inflation and would be worth (1,596/1.025^45) or the equivalent of 525 dollars in today's dollars after inflation. So, think about it… For every 50 dollars you spend, you are really using 525 dollars in "future money" when you are 70 years old. Are that meal and drinks worth 525 dollars?

Now let's think about these calculations a little bit deeper. Let's say you decide to put away those 50 dollars each month for your full first year of work. That would be 50 x 12 or 600 dollars saved for this year when you are 26 years old. Or, approximately 6,300 "future 70-year-old" dollars saved (525 dollars x 12) after inflation. How long would it take to save the same amount of money at 50 years old (at peak earnings age) at 50 dollars per month? It would be the following calculation for 7 years of savings:

600+ (600*1.08/1.025)+ (600*1.08^2/1.025^2)+(600*1.08^3/1.025^3)+ (600*1.08^4/1.025^4) + (600*1.08^5/1.025^5) +(600*1.08^6/1.025^6) + (600*1.08^7/1.025^7) or 5,823 dollars after 7 years.

If you add another year of saving at 50 dollars per month you come up with an additional (600*1.08^8/1.025^8) for a total of 6,734 dollars at 8 years.

In other words, you would need to save between 7-8 years at 50 dollars per month when you are 50 years old to come up with an approximate total of 6,300 dollars of future money. This compares to the spry age of 26 when you only need to save 50 dollars per month for one year in order to come up with the same amount at 70 years old. So, the bottom line is that even though you will be making a lot more in the future, your future dollars are nowhere near as powerful as today's dollars. You may be making 10 times as many dollars, but each dollar earned may be 7-8 times less powerful. This is a good reason alone to start investing today.

ANOTHER REASON WHY INVESTING IS SO IMPORTANT NOW- LOW PREVAILING INTEREST RATES

It turns out that interest rates are still very low in the year of this book's publication- 2017. And, there is no guarantee that interest rates are going to return to the high single digits or above for a very long time. So, in retirement, you need a significantly larger nest egg than you would have needed 10, 20, or 30 years ago. Today, you can get a maximum "safe" interest rate of 3.5-4% on instruments such as municipal bonds. And the 30-year Treasury bond, another safe investment, yields only 3%. So, if you want a guaranteed income when you get older, you may need to save twice or three times as much as many years ago when the same interest rates would have been 6 percent, 7 percent, or more. Think of it this way- today you have a million dollars, you only collect 35-40 thousand dollars per year. 30 years ago with that same million dollars collecting interest at 10 percent, you would have had a hundred thousand dollars per year. That's a really significant difference in the potential quality of retirement. It behooves all of us in the year 2016 to become really conscientious savers/investors.

The Importance of Basic Investing Habits

I would also argue that as human beings, we tend to do many things habitually. We brush our teeth, go to work, take a shower, etc. If you don't develop those habits at an early age, it may never become part of your routine. I would say that the same idea goes for putting away investment money on a monthly basis. Those radiology residents that don't start investing on a monthly basis early in their career are much less likely to do the same when they are further on in their career. You are likely to want to spend without thinking about the possibility of your future if it is not a habit. Also, you need to develop a comfort level with how to invest. If you don't start, you will not know the basics and be less likely to contribute. And most importantly, believe it or not... We all can't work forever!!! Who knows how much will be left in the Social Security trust fund by the time you retire?

What's the upshot?

So, the crucial factors of compounding and low prevailing interest rates are really important reasons to start saving that extra 50 dollars or whatever you have at the end of the month in an investment account. Start making a concerted effort to plug away at your retirement account so that it becomes a habit of investing monthly for the rest of your life and you feel comfortable doing so. It's not just 50 dollars per month or 600 dollars per year. It's a nice gift of 6300 dollars per year for your 70-year-old birthday and it's not just chump change. For your sake and for your retirement's sake, I recommend that you start putting away money for investment, no matter how small, right now!!!

(1) http://pages.stern.nyu.edu/~adamodar/New_Home_Page/datafile/histretSP.html

● ● ●

THE DISTINCTION BETWEEN INVESTING AND savings is not trivial. It can lead to the loss of thousands of dollars if the two ideas are misused or confused. Since most residents do not have business backgrounds, I'm pretty sure there is a high percentage of radiology residents that do not understand the difference between investments and savings. So, I am going to simply define each, show why it is so important to understand the distinction, and then go into more detail about what constitutes savings. Due to time constraints, I will leave a full investigation of types of investments and how to invest to another chapter. (Let's make it part 2!!!)

SAVINGS VS. INVESTMENT DEFINITION

First off, the definitions. Savings are short-term instruments for keeping/holding onto money, usually for less than 5 years. Investments are long-term instruments for creating wealth.

Why is this distinction so important? If you are putting investment money into savings, you are losing out on the opportunity cost of making high interest/capital appreciation on your money. Likewise, if you are putting savings money into investments, you are substantially increasing your risk on money that you need, or risking the need for capital preservation.

WHAT CAN HAPPEN IF YOU TREAT AN INVESTMENT AS SAVINGS?

Let's start with a thought experiment: putting investment money into savings. Imagine you have 1,000 dollars that you can afford to put away for a long period of time. Logically, what is the safest way to utilize this money? Many would say put it in a FDIC insured bank account, possibly a certificate of deposit. Wrong, wrong, wrong!!! In fact, the risks to this money become substantial.

What can you get on a 5-year CD? Maybe 2 percent, if lucky. Now, what is the current inflation rate? It is about 1.86%. (There is handy calculator called the CPI calculator (1) that you can use to calculate the yearly inflation rate). So, you decide to put the 1,000 dollars into a 5-year CD. At the end of 5 years, you collect the interest which is 1,000 * (1.02^5-1) or about 104 dollars. But wait. The government has to take its fair share of the interest with taxes. Taxes on interest are pretty much the same as your regular income taxes. So, let's say you are in the 25% tax bracket and you have a 3% state tax on interest, you are now left with 104*(1-(0.25+0.03)) or around 75 dollars. So, you have 1,000+75 or 1,075 dollars after taxes and interest. However, what are 1,075 dollars really worth 5 years later? Here, we need to take the prevailing Consumer Price Index (CPI) number (for simplicity sake we will assume it is 1.86% each year, the current CPI rate). So we take the 1075 dollars and divide that by the following number- 1.0186^5, or 1.097, the total effect of inflation over 5 years. So how much is the 1,075 dollars in 5 years worth in present dollars- that would be 1,075/1.097 or 980 dollars. Think about it. The 1,000 dollars that you put into the 5-year cd is really worth only 980 dollars when you take it out. That's a really raw deal. Your money will be guaranteed to be eaten up by taxes and inflation in this low-interest environment over a long period of time. Don't put your investment money into savings!

WHAT CAN HAPPEN IF YOU TREAT SAVINGS AS AN INVESTMENT?

All right, let's take the opposite situation. You have a 12-year-old car that is in its last 10-20 thousand miles. You decide to take those 1,000 dollars and put it into an S & P index fund to save for a car over the next three years when you think you will need one. It happens to be the year 2006. What happened to the S & P index fund between Jan 1, 2006, and Jan 1, 2009? It fell by 35%. And, you need that money to afford to buy a car in 2009. So, now you only have 1,000*(1 -0.35) or 650 dollars in 2009. You may now not be able to afford to buy the car you wanted. Even worse, you may have to take that 650 dollars and use it to buy your car. Think about it. Subsequently, in the period of time afterward from 2009-2016, the stock market went up about 158 percent. That same original 1000 dollars you would have put into the index fund would have been worth over 68% more in 2016 or (1.68*1000) 1,680 dollars if you kept it invested. Or those 650 dollars that you used in 2009 would have been worth 1,680 dollars in 2016. Hmmm... 650 dollars vs. 1,680 dollars only 7 years later, a striking difference.

The problem is you need to use your savings when you need to use your savings. You have little control over timing. Often times, you will wind up selling your investment at a low point, meaning that you will lose the potential capital appreciation of your initial investment. Any money that you need over the short term should not be placed in an instrument with significant risk. Never put your short-term savings into an investment!

Types of Savings

So now you understand why it is important not to take too many risks with your money for short-term needs. But, there are many options. For the uninitiated, this can seem daunting. I think of it as a multilayered approach. Let's put the type of savings into two different types of buckets: money you may need for something immediately (100 percent liquid savings) and money you don't need immediately but you will need in the short-term future (up to 5 years later).

Liquid Savings Accounts

Which savings instruments are 100 percent liquid? Checking accounts, money market accounts, FDIC insured savings accounts and money market funds.

I will begin with checking accounts, probably the most familiar. You can establish a checking account at almost any bank or credit union, online or in person. And, you probably have one already. It usually issues almost no interest but allows instant access anytime. I personally have a checking account with a local branch, but an online checking account is likely ok for most people.

Money market funds are safe heavily diversified accounts that invest in large numbers of short-term notes that usually return a nominal amount of interest. They are common at brokerage houses. Some allow you to write checks against the account. They are a good place to park cash temporarily, often as an instrument to buy investments at some point. But, it is safe enough to be considered 100 percent liquid and a savings instrument.

Money market accounts are available at banks and usually also allow instant access to your money, but for a limited number of times per month. You can typically write checks against the account. The advantage of this account: they usually provide a higher interest rate than a checking account and it is also FDIC insured. I would tend to put money in this account for less frequent and larger expenses. Also, if someone steals your checking account information, it provides an additional level of security. Not all of your money will be in the most readily accessible checking account.

And, there are FDIC insured savings accounts. They are very similar to money market accounts but usually don't allow direct checks against them. You can move money instantaneously in and out of them electronically. Similar to money market accounts, they provide a higher level of interest. I personally recommend looking into online savings accounts because they tend to issue a higher interest rate since these online banks don't have the fixed costs of local branches. This sort of account can be used to save for short-term larger purchases.

Less Liquid Savings Options

Let's say you don't need instant access to your money, but you do need it sometime in the near future. These options provide a slightly higher interest rate with the main intention of capital preservation and not capital appreciation. Remember, these savings instruments should not be seen as means to make tons of money, but rather a means to be able to pay for important/necessary expenses. Many residents have not had much experience with these options. Nonetheless, they are really important to understand. What are some of these options? The main ones are bank CDs, brokerage CDs, short-term treasuries, "investment grade" short-term municipal bonds, and "investment grade" short-term corporate bonds.

So let's talk about bank CDs first. The type of bank CD I am talking about is a FDIC-insured bank CD only. This CD guarantees a fixed yearly interest rate for the duration of the time of the CD. You can use the principal and interest without penalty when the bank CD comes due. If you decide to cash in the CD prior to the due date, there is often an interest penalty that can vary with the bank offering the CD. Bank CDs often range from 3 months to 10 years and beyond. I would recommend using bank CDs in the range of 1 to 5 years. Why? Simply because very short-term bank CDs less than 1 year tend to offer lower interest rates than savings accounts and money market accounts with less liquidity. Bank CDs greater than 5 years break the golden rule of using savings accounts as an investment since a long-term CD tends to provide a much lower interest rate than what you can make in an investment.

Bank CDs are very useful for saving for items or events that you will definitely not need until a specified date since they offer a slightly higher interest rate than the standard savings account. You can also use them as a backup to an emergency account. It can be a place where you can save additional money with minimal penalty, if needed, with a higher interest rate.

I would also like to mention brokerage CDs as a similar sort of savings instrument. These CDs operate in a very similar fashion to a bank CD. The big difference is that you can buy these CDs at a brokerage and collect many different CDs from many different banks in one place. These CDs are very good for people that need a large amount of liquid money and don't want to have to worry about FDIC insurance limits for their money (250000 dollars- Not something for a typical resident to worry about!!!) You can also buy and sell the CDs prior to the due date at a loss or gain depending upon the changes in prevailing interest rates, something that you can't do easily with a bank CD.

Short-term Treasury notes are also another option as a safe short-term savings mechanism. The going interest rate is 1.31 percent for a five-year Treasury as of the date that the chapter is written. This interest rate tends to be somewhat lower than what you can get in a FDIC insured CD. So, I tend not to recommend them. But, it is also backed by the full faith of United States government and is unlikely to default. It is surely a safe means of capital preservation.

The final two less liquid savings options are closer to a hybrid between savings and investments since there is a slightly higher risk of default (meaning there is a theoretical risk that you won't get all your money back). These include investment grade short-term municipal bonds and corporate bonds.

For the typical radiology resident, municipal bonds are not the greatest deal because they tend to issue a lower interest rate than the other savings interest rates and you do not get the big benefit of the municipal bond, the ability of the instrument to be free from federal taxes. Most residents are in either the 15 or 25 percent federal tax bracket, so the advantage of buying these instruments is typically not there. You really need to be in higher tax brackets (above 35 percent) to take advantage of this instrument. At the current time, the median yield on a 5-year municipal bond ranges from 1.1-1.4 percent depending on the investment quality. If you figure, that the true interest rate including the tax benefit is somewhere around (1.1/0.85 to 1.4/0.75) or 1.29 to 1.86 percent, depending on the bond and your tax rate, there is not much benefit to this sort of bond and it has a very low but real risk of default.

Investment grade corporate bonds can be another interesting way to save money for a fixed period of time. The interest rates at the current time may be a touch higher than the typically high-interest bank CD. However, again there is a real but remote risk of a short-term high-quality company default. I would not recommend it at the current time.

Finally, I would briefly like to mention that there is also the option of short-term bond funds. The reason I don't like this option for savings is that there is a real risk of loss of principal (albeit not by that much typically), breaking the rule of using savings as an investment.

The Bottom Line

The biggest take home point is to remember savings are not investments and investments are not savings. Severe damage to your financial life can occur if you break this cardinal rule, even as a resident.

Also, there are multiple ways that you can put money into savings. For most residents, a checking account, money market account, and/or saving account make a lot of sense for the most liquid needs. In addition, I would recommend bank or brokerage CDs to those residents that don't need their savings for a slightly longer period of time (between 1-5 years) and want to accumulate a slightly higher interest rate.

Well, that's about it for a summary of the pitfalls of savings vs. investments and the basics of savings instruments. See you back here in the next chapter for part 2 of this series!

(1) https://data.bls.gov/cgi-bin/cpicalc.pl

APPENDIX E: INVESTMENTS VS. SAVINGS- A RESIDENT'S GUIDE PART 2

● ● ●

As a reminder, in the previous chapter, we went through the difference between savings and investments and talked about why the difference is so important with examples of using savings as an investment and investments as savings as a resident. We also discussed many different ways to put money away for savings. This is all encompassed in the last chapter called Investments vs. Savings- A Resident's Guide- Part 1. In this chapter, we are going to discuss what many residents are more excited about- what are the common options available for investing money as a resident? In particular, we will emphasize the usual individual types of investments available (stocks, bonds, mutual funds, and ETFs). This chapter is not going to include other sorts of alternative investments such as peer-peer lending, real estate, MLPs, etc. Also, I am not going to discuss the different overarching account types (IRAs, brokerage accounts, 401k, etc.). Both of these latter topics are grounds for another discussion as a full-blown article at a later point!!!

To make it easier to follow, I will divide the investment types into the following categories: stocks and bonds. I will give examples of each and examine which places are good to park your money as a radiology resident. Let's start with the best place to put your money for most residents: stocks.

Stocks

Before we begin with the types of investments, let's first address the definition of a stock. Simply put, a stock is a share or portion of a company.

An issued stock can be publicly traded or privately traded, meaning that some stocks can be traded on the public markets, like the New York Stock Exchange or the NASDAQ. Other private stocks/shares are not available for general public trading and you need to be an "insider" or in a private market to buy and sell available shares. For this discussion, we will emphasize publicly traded stocks because it is what is much more commonly available.

Some publicly traded stocks allow the investor to recover a percentage of a company's profits into something called a dividend. Dividends are often issued on a quarterly basis and can be either reinvested back into the shares of the company or can be taken by the individual investor as cash. Since dividends have been traditionally a large percentage of the annual return on investment, I would recommend the former strategy of reinvesting one's dividends.

When investing in stocks, there are two main ways to go about purchasing stocks, individually or in groups. As a radiology resident, most of you are not going to have much time to research and purchase stocks individually, so I would highly recommend following the strategy of buying groups of stocks. In fact, if you were going to pursue the individual stock picking strategy, I would wait until you finish your residency and fellowship when you can dedicate more time and resources toward this endeavor of "stock picking". For now, stick with the low maintenance plan, mutual funds, and ETFs.

Stock Mutual Funds/ETFs

Stock mutual funds and ETFs (exchange traded funds) are groups of stocks that you can buy and sell, usually run by a portfolio manager. The price of the mutual fund is set at one time, at the end of the day. And, the mutual fund can only be bought or sold at the end of the day price.

The portfolio manager usually charges a fee to maintain the portfolio of a mutual fund. Sometimes it's baked into the price of the mutual fund. Other times, there is an additional fee called a load. Sometimes the load is added to the purchase price of the mutual fund on the "front end", meaning that the fee is added at the initial purchase time. Other times, it is added at the "back end", meaning that the fee is added when you sell the mutual fund. That fee can range as high as 5% of the value of the purchase price. I would tend to stay away from mutual funds that charge a load because it erodes the potential earnings from the mutual fund investment. You essentially have to subtract the 1-5% load from the annual earnings that you make from the fund, so it is possible that you can actually have a loss for the year in the fund even though the fund has made money!

On the other hand, an ETF price changes continually throughout the day and can be bought and sold at any time. Whenever you buy or sell an ETF, typically you have to pay a brokerage fee, which can be substantial relative to the amount that you are buying at a resident's salary level. If you want to buy 50 dollars of an ETF and the brokerage fee is $7.95, you are being charged (7.95/50*100) or 15.9 percent, an exorbitant amount. For this reason, if you are going to buy an ETF, it only makes sense at a resident level if you can afford to buy it in 1 thousand dollar increments or more. I typically like ETFs overall more than mutual funds because of the flexibility of buying and selling these instruments at any time during the given day, if needed. But, you have to be able to put enough money into the ETF for it to make sense at a resident level. So, your best bet is to purchase a no-load mutual fund.

What types of mutual funds or ETF should you buy?

My suggestion is to stick to index funds. Index funds are funds that follow an index such as the Standard and Poors 500, the Russell 2000, and so on. They are groups of stocks that are widely followed and generally have a theme. They may follow large capitalization stocks, small capitalization stocks, international stocks, value stocks, growth stocks, and more. Index funds are not actively managed portfolios, meaning that the manager just follows whatever the index does when it comes to buying or selling stocks within the index. For this reason, the fees on these funds tend to be significantly lower because the manager does not have to make these decisions on his/her own and tends to trade a lot less.

On the other hand, actively managed mutual funds allow the portfolio manager to buy and sell stocks on his/her own. Therefore, these managers are paid a higher managing fee. These funds also tend to have higher turnover costs from more frequent buying and selling within the fund and that may erode the original purchase price of the mutual fund. For these reasons, I would tend to stick with the index fund at your stage as a resident.

Diversification

I would also recommend that you should diversify your mutual fund holdings, whether you decide to purchase a mutual fund or an ETF. Diversification allows you to profit from upswings in any given investing theme when money is being made and prevents you from losing a lot when one theme is not doing so well. What does that mean? When you are buying a mutual fund or ETF, make sure to buy one that invests in large cap stocks (like the S & P 500), another that invest in mid-capitalization stocks, another that invests in small capitalization stocks, and another that invests in international stocks. Sometimes large capitalization stocks perform the best and others times it is small capitalization stocks. And likewise, sometimes any one of these options will perform poorly. Therefore, the upswings and downswings will be more muted (otherwise called reducing volatility). Typically, it is more tolerable to have losses that are not exorbitant!!!

Individual Stocks

Buying and selling individual stocks takes time, research, and a desire to do so. Stocks need to be monitored continually because news may come out about a company that may change the reason you bought the company. And, you may not be available to buy or sell the stock at that time, especially as a resident. So, it generally does not make sense for the radiology resident to purchase individual stocks. I think concentrating on a prospective career and becoming the best radiologist possible would better serve most residents. It will have a much higher payoff than taking the time to invest in individual stocks. When you have finished training, you can decide for yourself whether to invest in individual stocks if you have the inclination.

BONDS

What are bonds? Bonds are essentially loans that are taken out by an entity that is scheduled to be repaid with interest to the buyer. The federal government, municipalities, corporate entities, or private persons can issue bonds.

In the current environment, the prevailing interest rates are extremely low and the interest provided to the buyer is very low. So, returns on investments are muted. When interest rates start to rise, your bond becomes less valuable due to erosion from interest rate risk and inflation. When interest rates decline, the value of your bond holding increases. It is very unlikely that we will see interest rates go much lower given the innately low rate at the present time. So, you are investing in an asset class without much upside. Granted, the potential to lose your initial capital investment is lower than a stock if you hold a bond to maturity (the due date). But the potential to have capital appreciation is also significantly lower and risks of inflation eroding your investment become substantially higher. Also, when you are young the potential for compounding your interest is much higher with a stock than a bond over a long period of time. For these reasons, I would stay away from investing too much of your money in bonds at the present time, perhaps no more than 5-10 percent, if that.

SHORT, INTERMEDIATE, AND LONG DATED BONDS

Time to bond maturity is a very important concept that all investors/residents should understand. When you invest in a bond or bond fund that invests in bonds that expire a long time from the present date, the value of your holding is much more volatile than a short term dated bond. If you think about it, it makes a lot of sense. When interest rates rise, your bond becomes less valuable because your interest is now lower compared to other new bonds out on the market. Also, the maturity date is far away and you have years and years of interest that will accumulate over time. So, now those years and years of interest are less valuable as well. With a short term bond or bond fund/ETF, you only have potentially a few years or months at your current interest rate, so the value will not change as much from face value. Therefore, in rising rate environments, long-dated bonds are usually not as valuable investments.

FEDERAL GOVERNMENT BONDS

These bonds are backed by the federal government and are the safest bonds in terms of default rates. (Missing interest payments or principal payments) It is significantly less likely for the United States government to default than a municipality or corporation. Due to a lower risk profile, these bonds are issued at a lower rate than other entities. Bond maturity length range from a few months to 30 years. There are a variety of different types of federal bonds including Treasury bills (short-term notes with maturity dates less than one year), notes (intermediate notes with maturity dates between 1-10 years), and bonds (long-term notes with maturity dates greater than 10 years). Treasury notes and bonds issue interest every 6 months. There are also treasury inflation protected securities (TIPS). These bonds adjust interest rates based upon the consumer price index. And, there are federal savings bonds. These bonds do not offer coupons/interest payments and are redeemed at the maturity value.

MUNICIPAL BONDS

Individual municipalities including local, county, and state governments back municipal bonds. The interest on these bonds is usually not taxed by the federal government. They also tend to offer lower coupons/interest payments than other types of bonds. So, they are usually more advantageous to investors in higher tax brackets (usually not a resident!!!). Although they have a significant role in a radiology attending's portfolio, at your stage of the game, I would generally avoid this group of bonds.

CORPORATE BONDS

Corporate bonds are backed by individual corporations and vary widely in quality and duration. Corporate bonds have a real default rate (some companies go out of business!!!), but they can potentially be a good investment. Corporate bonds range in quality from investment grade to junk bonds, based upon the likelihood of default. Interest rates are typically higher than government issued bonds.

BOND MUTUAL FUNDS/ETFS

What are bond mutual funds and ETFs? These investing instruments are very similar to stock mutual funds and ETFs. They are groups of bonds that are being invested by a large entity such as a brokerage and are run by a portfolio manager. Just like stock mutual funds and ETFs, bond mutual funds are valued at the end of the day and can only be bought and sold at the end of the day. ETFs can be continually bought and sold throughout normal business hours. Portfolio managers charge fees for bond ETFs and mutual funds just like stock mutual funds. Again, avoid funds with loads because they can significantly reduce your return on investment.

Unlike stock mutual funds and ETFs, bond mutual funds and ETFs may not necessarily be better than individual bonds held to maturity. The reason is that bonds can be bought and sold at different prices from the face value of the bond (a loss or gain) when you are invested in a mutual fund or ETF. So, the price of the bond fund can be less than the price at which you originally bought the fund. On the other hand, if you hold your own individual bond to maturity, you are guaranteed to get the face value back (as long as the bond does not default!). Bond funds and ETF also continually take money from the sold and maturing bonds and reinvest the proceeds into new bonds. These new bonds can have a higher or lower interest rate than the original purchase depending on market conditions. During times of rising rates, you may notice that your bond fund rates will rise and the prices will decline. During times of falling rates, you will experience decreasing interest rates and increasing prices of your bond fund/ETF.

Many plans only allow the purchasers to buy bond mutual funds and not individual bonds. So, my recommendation would be to find a diversified bond fund that invests in federal government, international government, and corporate bonds with a nice mix of different maturity dates. In this sort of low-interest rate environment, you may want to refrain from investing too much in this sort of instrument, especially as a young resident with years and years ahead of you.

INDIVIDUAL BONDS

On the other hand, individual bonds typically have a fixed interest rate that is determined at the time of purchase. And at the time of maturity, you will get the face value back of the bond. For this reason, individual bonds are not a bad choice if you have enough money to diversify and buy a few treasuries and corporate bonds of varying quality and duration. The problem is that residents often do not have enough capital to make purchasing multiple individual bonds a viable option. So, for most residents consider the mutual fund/ETF option if you decide to invest in bonds. But remember... as a resident, only a minimal amount should be invested in this category due to lack of capital appreciation with respect to inflation.

WHAT DOES THE RESIDENT INVESTOR REALLY NEED TO KNOW IN THE END?

Stocks and bonds are the mainstays of resident investing. Due to the long road ahead for residents, you should be concentrating on investment capital appreciation and not capital preservation. So, look into holding a lot more stock related assets than bond related assets (probably not much more than 5-10%). If you are going to buy stocks, buy diversified index mutual funds covering the different types stocks- large caps, intermediate caps, small caps, and foreign stocks. If you are going to buy bonds, most residents should buy a diversified fund of treasuries and corporates with widely varying maturities. Residency is a time to learn about your prospective field, so make sure to automate your investments as much as possible by putting money away on a regular automated basis (weekly, biweekly, or monthly). Don't forget- your dollar is much more powerful when you are young, so it is important to invest and stay in the game!!!

● ● ●

UNLIKE OTHER COUNTRIES, MASS TRANSPORTATION is not available in all parts of the United States due to infrastructure issues and spread out spaces. For this reason, many medical residents may face the decision of buying or leasing a car during residency. It may not be such a simple question. In fact, several times my residents have asked that I write a post on this subject matter on radsresident.com. So, I will first define what it means to lease a car and then I will explain how I would make a decision to buy versus lease a car with multiple thought experiments and comparisons.

WHAT IS A CAR LEASE?
A car lease is a hybrid between buying and renting a car. It allows the lessor to spend a portion of the entire cost of the car over a fixed period, usually with the option to buy the car at the end of the lease period at a depreciated amount. Monthly payments are typically less than buying a car since the whole cost of the car is not included in the price. The lease cost usually includes the depreciating cost of the car and monthly interest. Additional fees included in the monthly bill are a cost for going over a fixed limit of miles and additional insurance costs above and beyond a typical owned car. Often times, the lessor also will put down a nominal fee at the beginning of the lease period as well. Bottom line- the process of leasing a car lets the lessee enjoy a more expensive car than he/she could

typically afford with lower monthly payments. But, the big question is- do they come at a significant cost?

Examples of Buying Vs. Leasing Cars

Whenever I make a financial decision, I always like to make a mental picture of the different financial possibilities by using thought experiments. Otherwise, it can be hard to understand the subtleties of the different arrangements. So, I am going to do just that with a typical car. I am going to assume the car costs about 30,000 dollars and that we are going to buy or lease the car over a 3-year period. Cars can be less costly if bought used, but for the point I am trying to make in this article, buying or leasing a new versus used car should not change the final conclusions. In my first example, I am going to assume that we are going to hold the car we bought over 10 years and compare that to the costs of leasing for three years and buying out the lease after the 3 year period is over. So, let's do just that...

Scenario 1- Buying and Holding for 10 Years Vs. Leasing And Buying Out A Lease

Let's say the interest rates are 3% on both the 3-year loan for a new car and the lease. And, we are going to put down a nominal amount on the car on both the car purchase and lease- say 2,000 dollars on both. So, what are the monthly and total costs of buying a car over the entire period? To determine that, I am going to use one of my favorite financial programs in the world- a very simple amortization calculator on the web from Bret Whissel called <u>Amortization Calculator</u>.(1) So, the monthly payments over a 3 year period on a bought car after the nominal down payment is approximately 814 dollars for a total amount of the 3 year loan of approximately 29,313 dollars. The total cost of buying the car will be 2,000+29,313 dollars or 31,313 dollars total.

How does this compare to the monthly payments on a 3-year car lease? Let's do the calculations. One of my favorite rules for determining depreciation of a car that approximates reality is the rule of 10+9+8+7+ 6+5+4+3+2+1. Each year that you own the car over a period up to 10 years can be approximated by taking the number of years that you own the car, adding the numbers from highest to lowest for that period of time and then dividing by the total of the rule (55). So in this case, the amount of depreciation over 3 years would be 10+9+8/55 or 49%. Alternatively, you can use a slightly more accurate calculator such as this one from <u>Money-zine</u> (2) and come up with a depreciation percentage, which would be approximately 39%. For the sake of "accuracy", we will use the more accurate calculator. The initial total lump sum of 3-year monthly payments is going to be (0.39) (30,000-2,000) or 10,920 dollars without interest. Calculating interest at a 3% rate and using the amortization calculator, the monthly payments are going to be 317.57 dollars and the total sum of payments over the 3-year period will be 11,433 dollars.

According to the calculations, the residual value of the car is now going to be 30,000*(1-0.39) or 18,300 dollars. Remember the 2,000 dollars that you put down on the car does not contribute to principal/cost basis of the vehicle. So, let's finance the payments of the residual value over 3 years again at 3%. The monthly payments this second time around for buying the car out of the lease are going to be about 532 dollars and the sum of the payments are going to be 19,159 dollars. So, the total cost of the vehicle after leasing and then buying out the lease are going to be 2,000+11,433+19,159 dollars for a total of 32,592 dollars, not including additional leasing fees. The additional cost for leasing and then buying out the car to get the lower payments vs. buying over a 3-year period is 32,592-31,313 or 1,279 dollars total, a mild difference.

Scenario 2- Buying and Holding Vs. Continually Leasing for 10 Years

In the second example, I am going to look at the costs of leasing when you do not buy out the lease, continually leasing cars every 3 years over a 10-year period, and compare that to buying a car and holding it for 10 years. So as in our first example, the initial cost of leasing the car over a three-year period is going to be 11,433+2,000 dollars. Let's assume you are going to do that three and a third times over a 10-year period. So, our total costs for leasing a car continually over the 10 year period would be 3.33*(11,433+2,000) or 44,732 dollars.

For comparison, when we buy and hold a car for 10 years, there are likely going to be increased repair costs for keeping a relatively older car. Let us then go ahead and add an additional 500 dollars per year in repair costs after the initial 3 years of the loan for buying the car. We will add that to the former loan price in the prior example or 31,313+(7*500) or 34,813 dollars. So, the additional cost for leasing a car continually over a 10 year period compared to buying a car and holding for 10 years would be 44,732-34,813 dollars or 9,919 dollars, almost a third of the price of a car!!!

SCENARIO 3- BUYING AND HOLDING VS. CONTINUALLY LEASING FOR 10 YEARS WITH TAX DEDUCTIONS

In the third example, I am going to assume that the resident is going to be moonlighting and is able to deduct the depreciated value of the car from his/her total income on an annual basis at the rate of 25%. We will again compare the costs of releasing a car every 3 years for 10 years and comparing that with buying a car and holding it for 10 years. Assuming you can deduct the depreciation from your salary, the new costs of leasing a car would be [11,433 (1-0.25) +2,000]*3.33 or 35,214 dollars over a 10 year period. The additional cost for leasing a car continually over a 10-year period in this situation would be 35,214- 34,813 dollars or 401 dollars, a bit more reasonable...

SCENARIO 4- BUYING AND SELLING OVER 10 YEARS VS. CONTINUALLY LEASING OVER 10 YEARS

In this example, I am going to compare what it would cost to buy and sell a new car every three years assuming a 30,000-dollar price tag for a 10-year period without leasing vs. the cost of leasing cars over a 10-year period.

Most residents don't like to have the hassle of constantly buying and selling cars, but it would be interesting to do the comparison with leasing over the same period of time. So, let's do the calculations.

Based on our initial scenario, the cost of buying the car over each 3-year period would be 31,313 dollars. So let's assume we can sell the car over each 3 year period for 31,313 dollars*(1-0.39) or the depreciated value of 19101 dollars. So, the cost over a 10 year period would be 3.33*(31,313-19,100) dollars for a total of 40,669 dollars. The additional cost for leasing cars over 10 years vs. buying and selling cars over a 10-year period would, therefore, be 44,732-40,669 dollars or 4,063 dollars, a moderate difference.

Scenario 5- Buying and Selling Over 10 Years vs. Continually Leasing Over 10 Years With Deductions

Finally, let's compare the cost of leasing over 10 years with the ability to deduct the depreciated lease value from your taxes compared to the cost of buying and selling cars every three years for a total of 10 years. The calculations were performed in several of the scenarios above, making these calculations easy. So, the total in this situation would be 35214 dollars for leasing and 40,669 dollars for buying and selling over 10 years. This is the one scenario where it would be less costly to lease for a total savings of 40,669-35,214 dollars or 5,455 dollars total.

What Can We Conclude Based on These Scenarios?

We have crunched all the numbers and what can we conclude? The starkest difference under all these scenarios is the difference between continually leasing a car over 10 years and buying a car and holding it for 10 years. You would theoretically save a total of 9,919 dollars over a 10 year period if you buy and hold a car, approximately 1/3 the value of the car. That's a lot of money!!!

If you are able to deduct the depreciated value of the car from your income, then leasing a car every 3 years for a 10 year period will be only at a slightly increased cost compared to holding on to a car for 10 years. If you like new cars, this proposition can make some sense.

Finally, the finances are almost always in favor of buying a car except for the one situation where you have to decide between leasing a car every 3 years for 10 years and buying and selling a car every 3 years for 10 years with the condition that you can deduct the depreciated lease value from your taxes because you are an independent practitioner/moonlighter/consultant. This would be a highly unusual situation.

Final Thoughts

Make sure to always crunch the numbers based upon your own inputs (these may vary slightly from mine). But, for most of you residents out there, if you need a ride to work and must have a car- go buy a car if you can and avoid the lease. A lease will put you a bit behind the eight ball over your initial working years, especially when it is most crucial to get rid of your student debt and begin your savings/investments. On the other hand, if you are able to deduct the depreciated value of the car from other self-employment income, then an argument can be made to lease instead of buy. And finally, if you are in the fortunate situation of being able to walk to work every day, perhaps you can do without a car altogether and really save some money!!!

(1) http://bretwhissel.net/cgi-bin/amortize

(2) http://www.money-zine.com/calculators/auto-loan-calculators/car-depreciation-calculator/

CHIEF AUTHOR BARRY JULIUS, MD, attended the Albert Einstein College of Medicine, completed his diagnostic-radiology residency at Brown University's Rhode Island Hospital, and completed his fellowship at the Harvard Joint Program in Nuclear Medicine. He is certified by the American Board of Radiology and the American Board of Nuclear Medicine.

Dr. Julius has been a radiologist at Saint Barnabas Medical Center in Livingston, New Jersey since 2006. Since 2009, he has served as associate program director for the Saint Barnabas Medical Center diagnostic-radiology residency, and he has been a partner at Imaging Consultants of Essex. He has been the editor in chief of radsresident.com since 2016.

Daniel Choe, DO, Leonard Morneau, MD, and Danny Nahl, MD, are associate authors. Together, the authors made it their mission to address the specific application, lifestyle, and career issues faced by radiology residents that fall outside the purview of typical medical training.

Made in the USA
Middletown, DE
05 October 2018